STARTING CALISTHENICS

A Beginner's Guide to Bodyweight Exercise & Mobility Training

Mo Saleem

Copyright © 2024 The Saleem Group

All rights reserved. No part of this book may be reproduced by any mechanical, photographic, or electronic process, or in the form of a phonographic recording; nor may it be stored in a retrieval system, transmitted, or otherwise be copied for public or private use—other than for "fair use" as brief quotations embodied in articles and reviews—without prior written permission of the publisher. All efforts have been made to ensure this publication provides accurate and authoritative information regarding the subject matter covered. It is sold with the understanding that the publisher is not engaged in rendering medical services. If you require medical advice, you should seek the services of a licensed professional. Disclaimer: The material contained in this book is for informational purposes only. The author and anyone else affiliated with the creation or distribution of this book may NOT be held liable for damages of any kind whatsoever allegedly caused or resulting from any such claimed reliance. Before beginning this or any fitness routine, it is recommended that you consult with a qualified physician for authorisation and clearance. If you have any problems with your health, you should seek clearance from a qualified medical professional. The information contained herein is not intended to, and never should, substitute for the necessity of seeking the advice of a medical professional. If at any time you feel pain or discomfort, stop immediately. Parts of this book contain advanced exercises that should not be attempted until you are ready.

*To Jim, whose indomitable spirit continues
to inspire. May he rest in peace.*

CONTENTS

Title Page
Copyright
Dedication
INTRODUCTION: START HERE — 1
CHAPTER 1 - THE HOLY GRAIL OF FITNESS — 11
CHAPTER 2 - WHY EXERCISE WITH BODYWEIGHT — 19
CHAPTER 3 - CALISTHENICS DOWNSIDES — 33
CHAPTER 4 - THE TOTAL FITNESS PYRAMID — 42
CHAPTER 5 - SCULPTING SYMMETRY — 59
CHAPTER 6 - THE FIVE LAWS OF LIFTING — 73
CHAPTER 7 - CREATING ALIGNMENT PART I — 83
FREE GOODWILL — 121
CHAPTER 8 - CREATING ALIGNMENT PART II — 123
CHAPTER 9 - THE SIMPLE SIX EXERCISES — 153
CHAPTER 10 - BODYWEIGHT FITNESS STANDARDS — 182
CHAPTER 11 - CONSTRUCTING YOUR ROUTINE — 193
CHAPTER 12 - OKR GOAL SETTING — 213
CHAPTER 13 - THE MASTERY MENTALITY — 219
CONCLUSION - THE PATH AHEAD — 233
ABOUT THE AUTHOR — 236

INTRODUCTION: START HERE

"In the beginner's mind there are many possibilities. In the expert's mind there are few."

—SHUNRYU SUZUKI

I got everything wrong for the first five years of my fitness journey.

Picture this: It's early morning, and I'm in the gym, the clanking of weights echoing through the space. Sweat stinging my eyes as I load another plate onto the barbell. Bench press, squat, deadlift, barbell row, and overhead press—these were my bread and butter. I thought this was the path to strength, to power, to the ultimate body. I thought I was building something unbreakable.

Until I broke.

One morning, I'm grinding through my usual barbell back squats when suddenly, my right knee buckles. A flash of pain shoots through my leg, and before I know it, I'm on the ground, the barbell crashing onto the safety pins. My training partner rushes over, but I wave him off, forcing myself to stand. I laugh it off, telling myself it's nothing. And strangely, I can walk out of the gym just fine.

But when the morning sun creeps through my window the next day, I swing my legs out of bed—and collapse. My right knee refuses to bear weight. Pain shoots up my leg with every attempted step. The MRI scan confirms it: torn cartilage. My world shrinks to a set of crutches, doctor visits, and physiotherapy beds. And it's on one of those cold, sterile tables, with electrodes strapped to my leg, that the truth finally hits me like a sledgehammer.

I had been building my structure of strength upon a foundation of sand.

My mistake wasn't that I didn't work hard enough—it was that I had ignored the single most crucial element of fitness: mobility. I could bench press one and a half times my body weight, but what good was that when I couldn't even walk? The exercises I thought were strengthening me were actually holding me back. I realized then that true strength isn't just about muscles—it's about the architecture that supports them.

This book isn't about becoming the strongest person in the room. It's about how you can live a long, healthy, and active life by cultivating a body that can withstand the test of time. It's about learning how to build a fortress, not on sand, but on stone. Whether you want to climb mountains, chase after your kids, or just get out of bed without feeling like your joints are betraying you, it all starts with mobility.

Starting Calisthenics is a manual for building your body the right way—from the ground up.

Reclaiming Your Physical Potential

Towards the end of his life, a man I once knew watched the sunset with a gaze that spoke of chances never taken and adventures never had. His silent story, both literal and metaphorical, isn't unique to him. It's seen in the eyes of many who've walked through life without ever experiencing their true potential.

You've conquered peaks in your career and personal life, but mastering your health and fitness? That may feel like an arduous climb. Gym memberships, personal trainers, apps, diets, online programs, supplements — investments may have been made, but the return wasn't there. And maybe, deep down, you've started to wonder if this is it. If this is the best you can expect from your body—a constant battle against time, pain, and decline.

You've seen it happen, perhaps to your own father—a life of vigor slowly but surely overshadowed by age, leaving behind only memories of strength. That image haunts you. It's not just about losing your youthful appearance; it's the fear of losing your independence, the dread of a future where your body becomes a cage rather than a vessel for adventure.

But what if it didn't have to be that way? What if, instead of waging war against your body, you could learn to work with it? Imagine a future where your joints are supple, your movements are fluid, and every step you take feels like freedom. No more waking up in pain, no more skipping the activities you love out of fear of injury. Picture yourself effortlessly sprinting after your kids, hiking up trails without a second thought, or simply getting up from the floor without wincing. It's not about looking a certain way—it's about feeling alive in your own skin.

This isn't a pipe dream. This is the promise of calisthenics: building real world strength from the ground up, starting with the very foundation of your body—your joints. It's the path to reclaiming control, to not just adding years to your life but adding life to your years. Imagine shedding the doubts, the constant second-guessing, and finally feeling at home in your body, not as a passenger but as the driver. The aches, the frustration, the fear—they may have marked your journey, but they do not define its end. And with the right approach, you can rewrite your story.

The journey starts now.

Your Blueprint For Total Body Fitness

This book is a beginner's guide, but the fundamental principles you're about to discover remain relevant regardless of your fitness level. In fact, it's been my observation that those who have never worked out before, often have a distinct advantage over those who have been exercising for years.

For example, the push up (or press up) is often considered a beginner's exercise because we've been doing it since childhood. However, my coaching experience has taught me that many lack the basic body awareness and motor control to execute the movement correctly. Those who have been doing push ups the most often have the hardest time in learning the correct form and technique because their nervous system has integrated a specific, albeit incorrect, movement pattern. They must first unlearn bad habits before learning the correct ones. In contrast, beginners only have to learn, making their path to proper technique more straightforward.

Zen wisdom teaches us that in the beginner's mind, there are many possibilities, but in the expert's mind, there are few. If one's mind is already set in particular ways, there is no space for new ideas to take root. Think of it as an empty cup. If the cup is full, there is no room for more. Similarly, if you approach this book with a mind already filled with preconceived notions, you won't be able to absorb new methods and insights. As I attempt to pour my knowledge into you, I don't expect you to trust me blindly. All I ask is that you approach these concepts with an open mind and a willingness to learn.

Together, we'll break the chains of mainstream fitness and build a body not just for show, but for life. Through these pages, I will guide you, step-by-step, towards constructing a foundation of strong and stable joints that can support a magnificent physical structure of strength and beauty that lasts a lifetime. Whether you've struggled with joint pain, old injuries, or simply haven't found the right approach, you will get a blueprint to start getting stronger and moving better no matter your age or situation. You won't need fancy equipment, a gym membership, or hours of dedicated time. Just your body, a little space, and the desire to improve.

Here's exactly what you'll learn:

> **Joint Mobilization:** Discover how to properly condition your joints, preventing injuries and even healing past damage. I'll show you exercises that fortify your body's natural structure, making it resilient and capable of handling life's physical demands.
>
> **Building Complete Fitness:** Learn how to build strength, stamina, and flexibility with simple bodyweight exercises that target multiple muscle groups. You'll find out how to maximize your results with minimal time, so you can get stronger without dedicating hours every day.
>
> **Sculpting Your Body:** I'll teach you how to sculpt muscle proportions reminiscent of ancient Greek statues. This isn't about vanity—it's about having a physique that looks as good as it performs.
>
> **Mastering Consistency:** You'll cultivate a mindset that turns daily exercise into an effortless habit. No more starting and stopping; you'll develop the discipline to stay the course, unlocking the secret to

lasting results.

Imagine waking up each day feeling strong, balanced, and ready for anything. By the end of this book, you'll have the tools and knowledge to make this your reality.

Welcome to the start of your transformation.

From Pain To Purpose (Why I Wrote This Book)

Summer 2006.

The laughter at the pool wasn't just from the joy of splashing water—it was pointed at my chest. Kids cruelly mocked the jiggly "man boobs" that clung to me like unwelcome parasites. From that point of shame, my quest began — a journey that saw my body starved, sculpted, injured, and reborn.

Growing up, I battled with body image issues. I avoided wearing white t-shirts for fear of revealing my droopy chest. I skipped meals, jogged myself into exhaustion, and swallowed fat burner pills, desperately trying to mold myself into something I could be proud of. By the time I entered senior year of high school, I was malnourished—the only kid who was yet to hit puberty. Something had to change.

With insecurity at an all-time high, I joined a gym and started lifting weights. Being the shortest boy in class, my goal was to compensate by getting wide. I followed bodybuilding routines that I found online and was in the gym six times per week. I spent nearly my entire life savings at the time on supplements and ate six square meals a day. As fate would have it, puberty kicked in around that same time and I packed on decent muscle size within months thanks to the surge in testosterone.

People started treating me differently. I noticed a more respectful attitude from men. Glances from females turned into stares. Naturally, my confidence and self-esteem began to soar.

For the first time in my life, I finally felt comfortable in my own skin. Over the next five years, the gym was my refuge. Through sweat, pain, and dedication, I lived the highs of bodybuilding until my body sounded the alarm.

Lifting weights took a toll on my joints—not once, but twice—with the alarming 'pop' of torn knee cartilage. My right knee gave way under the weight of a heavy squat—torn lateral meniscus. A few years later, it was my left knee on the leg press—torn medial meniscus. Suddenly, the strong, confident persona I had built began to crumble as I found myself bedridden and battling with my sense of self-worth once again.

In the trenches of recovery, I reconsidered my entire approach to fitness. I dove into the study of human anatomy, experimented with yoga, stretching, and ancient healing techniques like Qi Gong. I spent time with physiotherapists, chiropractors, acupuncture practitioners, and anyone who could teach me about natural healing. And slowly, through a combination of disciplines that revolved around bodyweight exercise, I healed my injuries without surgery and built a body that was more resilient than ever before.

As my body healed, I began sharing my journey online. I started working with clients of all ages and fitness levels, from elite athletes to everyday people who had been let down by conventional fitness advice. One of those clients was Jim, a 79-year-old man with arthritis in every joint and a history of surgeries, including a spinal fusion. Doctors had written off his physical potential, but I saw something different. We worked together, and despite all the odds, Jim unlocked his first chin up—a feat he thought was impossible.

Then there was James, who had repeatedly injured himself lifting weights. Every few weeks, his lower back would seize up, leaving him in pain and frustration. Together, we identified the weak links and fortified his body through targeted mobility and strength work, making lower back pain a thing of the past. I worked with another client in his 70s who had never done a dip or chin up in his life. Yet, by focusing on mobility and foundational strength, he achieved those milestones for the first time, proving that age is just a number.

Even elite athletes faced challenges that traditional training couldn't solve. A world champion cyclist came to me unable to perform a single push up due to arthritic wrist pain. By adapting the principles of bodyweight training, we gradually rebuilt his strength, and he reclaimed his ability to do push ups, pull ups, and beyond.

These aren't just isolated success stories—they are proof that the principles in this book work, no matter your age or physical limitations. I've personally worked with hundreds of clients each with their own set of challenges, and I've seen firsthand how the right approach can change lives.

This book distills everything I've learned from my own journey and from coaching countless others. I wrote this book to share the lessons that took me years of trial, error, and recovery to learn, so you can avoid the mistakes I made and build a body that's truly strong, resilient, and up for everything you are.

What This Book Is (And What It Is Not)

Let's be frank. This book is not a magic bullet. If you're hunting for quick fixes, miracle shortcuts or a promise of miraculous transformation, this isn't the guide for you. The fitness world, as you've likely noticed, is cluttered with fads and flashy trends that promise instant results but deliver little more than disappointment. This book rejects such false promises.

Instead, what you'll find here is a commitment to understanding, discipline, and respect for your body's potential over a lifetime. This book is about equipping you with an understanding of calisthenics—rooted in principles honed through years of study, personal experience, and guiding others from all walks of life. It's about sustainable, long-term progress that prioritizes patience, persistence, and consistency.

You won't find any fluff here—just the distillation of essential knowledge and practices that work. But let's be clear: this requires your full engagement. You'll need to challenge yourself, break old habits, and commit to the journey. If you're ready to dive in, put in the work, and approach this with a long-term lens, then you're exactly where you need to be.

Are you prepared to redefine your relationship with exercise? To build a body that's not only strong but flexible and capable? If you're willing to invest in yourself—not for fleeting quick wins, but for the lasting transformation that comes from dedication—then let's get started.

As we turn the page to the first chapter, remember this:

The Holy Grail of fitness isn't found in restrictive diets, punishing gym routines, or the latest trendy gadgets. It's something much simpler, often overlooked, yet completely within your reach. It's time to rethink everything you know about exercise and honor the intricate design of your body. The foundation we lay here is crucial, and it all starts with a single, often-neglected element that could change everything for you.

Let's begin.

Grab These Free Implementation Resources

Don't just read this book—put it into action! You'll find implementation easier with these free resources. Go to this book's bonus page and get:

1. A cheat sheet for the book's key concepts.

2. An action guide to start burning fat for fuel.

3. A blueprint that outlines specific bodyweight fitness standards to aim for.

Head to CalisthenicsBook.com/bonus to get these free resources, or scan the QR code below:

CHAPTER 1 - THE HOLY GRAIL OF FITNESS

"Health is a crown on the well person's head that only the sick person can see."

—ANONYMOUS

His heart pounded against his chest, each beat echoing the urgency of his mission. With strong legs carrying him over the rugged Athenian landscape, Pheidippides, the ancient herald, was a symbol of pure, unadulterated fitness. His lungs filled with the fire of exertion as he surged forth on what was to become a legendary run, laying the foundations for what we call the marathon and Spartathlon races.

The fabled run from Athens to Sparta and back (covering about 240 kilometers or 150 miles in two days) was to request military assistance against the Persians when they landed in Marathon, Greece. After returning to Athens, Pheidippides ran to the battlefield near Marathon and then back to Athens again (covering about 40 kilometers or 26 miles) to announce Greek victory over the Persians.

As he arrived to deliver the news of victory - *"Nike!"* - Pheidippides collapsed and died. The very name that would come to symbolize triumph in the modern sportswear giant was birthed from a tale of victory that demanded the ultimate price.

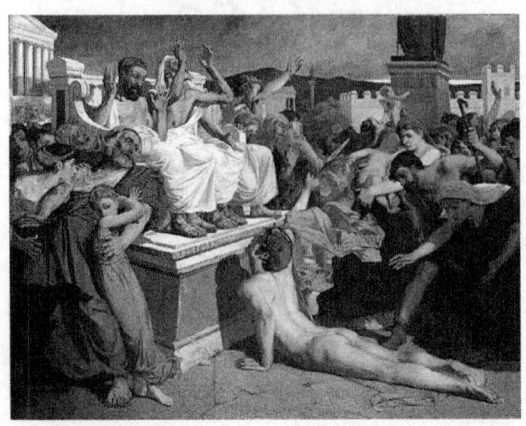

Painting of Pheidippides as he delivered news of Greek victory over the Persians before dying on the spot.

This story isn't just a piece of history; it's a warning. There's no doubt that Pheidippides had incredible fitness, but his health paid the ultimate price. We hear tales of his run and think of achievement, yet we miss the vital lesson about the balance between fitness and health.

And so, we must ask ourselves:

What is the true measure of fitness? Is it the capacity to run for miles until our last breath, or is it something more sustainable and profound?

As we stand upon the shoulders of the ancient herald's legacy, we encounter the central thesis of our quest:

The Holy Grail of fitness is longevity.

Living Long And Healthy

What is longevity?

The meaning we assign to words matters because it affects how we think about them. And how we think affects what we do. If we're thinking about words the wrong way, then we're likely to be doing the wrong things.

Throughout this book we will look at the origin of key words, observing how their meanings have shifted through time so that we can think about them the right way and, therefore, focus on doing the right things.

"The beginning of wisdom is the definition of terms."

—Socrates

Let's start by exploring the roots of *'longevity,'* a term that goes back to the Latin *'longus'* meaning *'long,'* and *'aevum,'* signifying *'age'* or *'lifetime.'* It's a concept that captures the length of life. However, the mere extension of life's timeline, as facilitated by modern advances in medicine and health, isn't our only criteria of success. For a life stretched long, absent of vigor and vitality, is like a book with many pages but scant story.

Chronological age—the count of years since birth—though easily quantified, is separate from biological age—the measure of how well our bodies function. This distinction is crucial because the ticking clock does not always reflect the rhythm of our biological function. Therefore, adding more candles to the birthday cake is only one part of *'longevity.'* The second part is to ensure that with each new candle, the light burns just as brightly.

Let us then define longevity as the combination of how many years we live, the *'lifespan,'* and how well we live during those years, the *'healthspan.'* This dual concept, lifespan coupled with healthspan, defines our pursuit—to live a long time with our health, strength and zest for life intact. In this narrative, the promise of a long life is about more than mere survival; it's about flourishing so that every additional year is matched with a body and mind capable of living it to the fullest.

As we continue, we'll explore how to nurture both our chronological selves and our biological beings so that each complements the other.

Metabolic Health Matters

What is health?

The roots of this word reach deep into history, coming from the Proto-Germanic *'hailitho,'* reflecting a sense of wholeness, and the Old Norse *'helge,'* meaning sacred or blessed. Old English embraced this with *'hælþ,'* tying it to a sense of being whole. The New Oxford American Dictionary defines health as *'the state of being free from illness or injury.'* But let's expand on this.

To be healthy is not just to be illness and injury-free, but to embody balance—especially in our metabolism. The dictionary defines metabolism as *'the chemical processes that occur within an organism in order to sustain life.'* These chemical processes are made up of anabolic and catabolic reactions. Anabolic reactions combine energy with smaller molecules to build larger molecules—like constructing a building brick by brick. Catabolic reactions break down larger molecules to release energy—like dismantling a building into bricks, wood, tiles etc. Both processes are essential but balance between the two is crucial.

Dr. Robert Lustig, world-leading endocrinologist and author of New York Times best seller *Fat Chance*, captures the significance of metabolic balance when he says that:

> "The simplest and cheapest surrogate for determining your health status is your waist circumference, which correlates with morbidity and risk for death better than any other health parameter. This is arguably the most important piece of information in your entire

health profile because it tells you about your visceral fat."

In other words, your waist measurement is a direct line to understanding the state of your metabolic health because it provides a glimpse into the store of visceral fat that surrounds the organs in your gut. Too much visceral fat is a sign of metabolic imbalance, with anabolic overshadowing catabolic reactions.

Armed with these insights, we now stand at the threshold of a new understanding. Fitness is not a sprint to maximum exertion, where we risk falling into the abyss of injury and illness. It is, instead, a mindful march towards the horizon of holistic health and vitality—a state characterized by a balanced metabolism.

Just as Pheidippides' historic run taught us the limits of endurance, our journey through this chapter has illuminated the path to true fitness—where the finish line is a long life lived with good health. Let us take with us the cautionary echo of his footsteps, a reminder to seek balance in every stride.

As we turn the page, we approach the next chapter where I make the case for why calisthenics is the supreme form of exercise in our quest towards ultimate health, fitness and longevity. Here, we will discuss how the simplicity of bodyweight exercise builds practical strength while protecting against injury. Prepare to explore how the gravity of your own mass is the only weight you need to sculpt a temple fit for the spirit of health and wellness.

Chapter Takeaways

- Longevity is our beacon, guiding us to a destination where the quantity of our years is matched by their quality. It is the combination of lifespan and healthspan, ensuring that we live not just longer, but healthier.

- Health goes beyond freedom from illness; it is a sacred balance that creates wholeness. To be healthy is to have a balanced metabolism, where the process of building up (anabolic reactions) and breaking down (catabolic reactions) remain in harmony.

- Fitness, while important, is not the sole measure of our well-being. It must be pursued with wisdom, ensuring it contributes to, rather than takes away from, our overall health.

- Visceral fat, as measured by waist circumference, stands as a simple yet profound indicator of our metabolic health status.

Success Check-In Exercise

Before we proceed with the rest of the book, let's check in with your current metabolic health.

Let your stomach hang loose in a neutral position and wrap a tape measure above your belly button in the area between your lowest rib and hip bone.

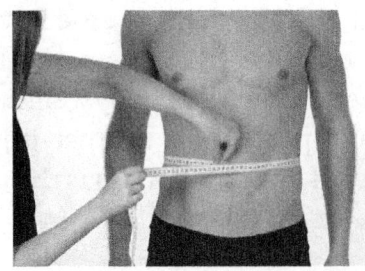

Your true waist measurement is the circumference of the area above your belly button rather than the size of pants you wear.

Take note of your current waist measurement in the following table:

	Current	Target	Difference
Waist Measurement	104 cm	72	32

Next, multiply your height by 0.45 to determine your target waist measurement and record it in the table as well.

Why 0.45? Because a waist measurement that is 45% or less of your height means that your waist is not carrying extra inches of fat, signifying metabolic balance. If your current waist is more than 45% of your height, then that is a sign of metabolic imbalance and the goal is to shed the extra inches.

Finally, subtract your target waist measurement from your current waist measurement to determine how many inches you have to lose.

If you don't have a tape measure handy, then you can approximate your current body fat by comparing it to the image below:

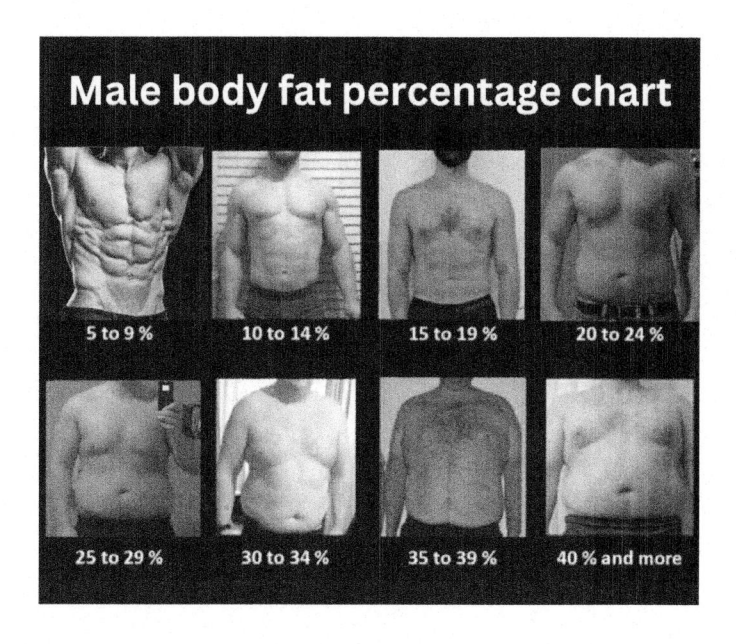

Take note of your current body fat percentage number versus your desired body fat percentage in the table below. With my clients, we aim for a body fat percentage less than 15%.

	Current	Desired
Body Fat Percentage	35-39	15.

CHAPTER 2 - WHY EXERCISE WITH BODYWEIGHT

"In nature, the human body doesn't need to move barbells or dumbbells around. Before it can move anything external at all, it has to be able to move itself around! It's sad to see that so many modern bodybuilders don't understand this fact. They train, first and foremost, to be able to move external objects."

—PAUL WADE

In the untamed wilderness of the Galápagos Islands, Charles Darwin looked upon the marvels of nature, a panorama of life's relentless pursuit of survival. Among finches and giant tortoises, Darwin developed his theory of evolution, a theory that would come to redefine our understanding of life itself.

It wasn't the brute strength of a beast, nor the higher intelligence of a primate that guaranteed survival, but rather an organism's ability to adapt to change. This principle of adaptability (Darwin's true definition of fitness) echoes through time to challenge our modern obsession with physical aesthetics. It strips down the fallacy that muscles sculpted to perfection under the shine of stage lights equate to the pinnacle of fitness. Instead, this principle speaks to a deeper, more intrinsic power—the ability to adapt, to move, to survive and thrive.

In the modern temple of fitness, where steel machines and mirrored walls stand as monuments to muscle, the essence of Darwin's theory is often lost. Here, in gyms scented with sweat, ambition and air freshener, the pursuit of a chiseled exterior has overshadowed the cultivation of the very adaptability that underpins survival — and indeed, our health.

The pageantry of bodybuilding, where the body is a canvas assessed on its looks rather than its ability to run, jump, and perform, exemplifies a major shift in mainstream fitness culture. This beauty contest of brawn has led to an obsession with form over function and appearance over ability.

As we stand on the shoulders of Darwin's legacy, we are reminded that the strongest or the smartest of species are not the ones that survive and thrive — it is those that can adapt to the ever-changing tapestry of life. And so, we come to the heart of our discussion on the benefits of calisthenics. It is a practice as old as humanity itself, a method that values the might of movement over the mirage of muscles.

Benefits Of Calisthenics

The New English Oxford dictionary defines calisthenics as *'gymnastic exercises to achieve bodily fitness and grace of movement.'* When we trace back to the roots of this word, calisthenics is actually a combination of the two ancient Greek words *'kallos,'* meaning beauty, and *'sthenos,'* meaning strength. That's what Socrates had in mind when he said that, "It is a shame for a man to grow old without seeing the beauty and strength of which his body is capable."

With modern context and ancient roots in mind, we arrive at the following definition:

Calisthenics is the practice of moving one's own body weight against gravity to sculpt a strong and beautiful physique that is capable of graceful movement.

In the symphony of physical training, calisthenics composes a melody that harmonizes the body's own weight with the pull of gravity.

Let's now look at the many benefits of bodyweight exercise—advantages that extend far beyond the surface and dive into the very essence of functionality.

Supple Strength: Strength Through Stretch

Calisthenics has a unique quality that sets it apart from other forms of training. This unique quality is that many bodyweight exercises require a high level of mobility, flexibility and joint stability to perform. For example, let's look at the single-leg squat below:

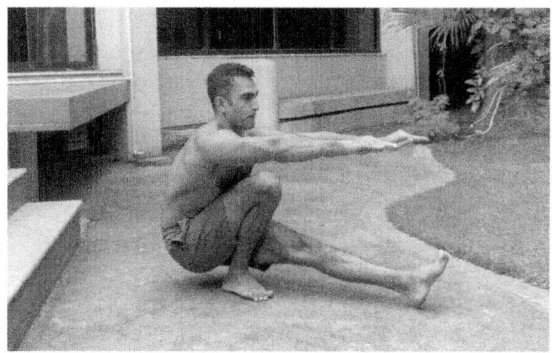

The single-leg squat is not a beginner's exercise and is therefore beyond the scope of this book. It is only being discussed here to explain the concept of supple strength.

A high level of lower-body strength is necessary to be able to squat on one leg, but strength is not the only requirement. Observe in the image above how the knee is fully bent and how the ankle bears the entire body's weight. The quad, knee and ankle tendons, while fully stretched, are forced to generate tension in order to keep the body upright. Also look at the stretch maintained by the hip and glute. The glute is stretched so far that the thigh is pressing against the torso. But while stretched, the glute and hip remain fully contracted in order to initiate the motion of pushing the body to stand back up again. This ability of muscles and tendons to contract and maintain tension while stretched is the definition of supple strength.

Supple strength is the harmonious combination of the ability to move, bend, and stretch (i.e. suppleness), with the capacity to exert force and maintain structural integrity (i.e. strength). It's not just about being strong or just being flexible; it's about having both qualities in balance. Supple strength is crucial for performing explosive movements (like jumping, sprinting, punching and kicking) with grace and control. Bodyweight exercises, like the single-leg squat, demand your muscles and tendons to stay strong while stretched, creating a more resilient and capable body.

> "Men are born soft and supple; dead they are stiff and hard. Plants are born tender and pliant; dead, they are brittle and dry. Thus whoever is stiff and inflexible is a disciple of death. Whoever is soft and yielding is a disciple of life."
>
> **—I Ching**

Mainstream fitness views flexibility as being able to hold stretched positions passively. Modern methods teach us to relax our muscles with conscious breathing as we get deeper into a stretch. Relaxing into a stretch does increase range of motion, but it's also potentially dangerous because injuries occur when ligaments, tendons, or soft tissues are overstretched.

The body has an in-built mechanism (called the myotatic reflex) that protects against overstretching by limiting range of motion. Traditional passive stretching desensitizes this reflex by replacing tension with relaxation in order to extend further. Supple strength challenges the concept of passive stretching by combining strength with flexibility. Building supple strength means that any increased range of motion is matched by the strength to control it, preventing injuries that arise from being stretched beyond controlled capacity.

With calisthenics, we're developing strength-led flexibility, or supple strength. This approach ensures that your body can safely generate force, even in stretched positions, making it a cornerstone of functional fitness.

Injury Prevention: Kinetic Harmony

My personal journey through fitness has had its fair share of struggles. Like many others, I've experienced significant injuries, which isn't uncommon in the weightlifting world. Issues like nagging shoulders or lower back pain are almost a given for seasoned weightlifters. Since transitioning to calisthenics, however, I've not only remained injury-free but have also healed prior joint injuries.

Take the push up, for example. Previously, I suffered with shoulder pain while doing barbell bench press. Having switched to full range of motion push ups, this pain has completely vanished. The beauty of bodyweight exercises lies in their natural tendency to encourage proper body alignment because the resistance is never heavier than your own body. This ensures that your skeletal structure aligns naturally, providing the most efficient and safe movement patterns. Calisthenics respects and enhances the natural function of your joints by strengthening them in harmony with your muscles, leading to a more balanced and resilient body.

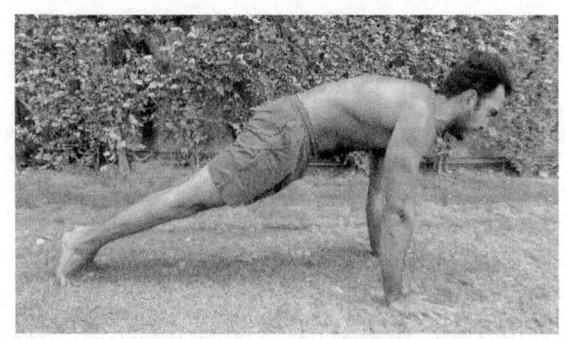

When performed properly, push ups stimulate the often neglected yet vital tissues that support our hands, fingers, wrists, forearms, elbows and shoulders.

A crucial point overlooked in modern training methods is the difference between muscle tissue and connective tissue adaptation. Muscle tissue can adapt to stimulus within 6-8 weeks while connective tissues can take 6 months to over a year. This is because tendons, ligaments, and fascia have a lower blood supply compared to muscle, meaning they receive fewer nutrients and less oxygen, which slows down their repair and adaptation process. With weightlifting, this can lead to a dangerous mismatch where muscle development outpaces connective tissue adaptation. When the muscle is strong enough to lift a certain amount of weight but the connective tissue is not, pain and injuries are around the corner.

Getting injured with calisthenics is possible, but not easy. With weightlifting, anyone can attempt to lift an amount they're not ready for by adding more weight to the bar. With bodyweight exercises, increasing intensity is more complex and cannot be rushed because we are unable to simply increase our body weight. Furthermore, advanced bodyweight exercises require months or years of skill development before they can even be attempted. This inherent limitation acts as a safeguard, ensuring that you only attempt exercises that your body is genuinely ready for. Compare this to barbell movements where any beginner can add 225 lbs (100 kg) to a bar and attempt to bench press with it.

What I've observed in working with clients and in myself is a testament to the protective nature of bodyweight exercise. Not only have my joints become stronger, but former aches and pains have disappeared.

Calisthenics is a holistic approach to fitness that respects and works with your body's natural mechanics, rather than against them.

Aesthetics: The Beauty Of Relative Strength

While functional ability is key, the desire for an attractive physique is a common and valid fitness goal. Modern methods emphasize appearance at the cost of ability, but with calisthenics these two aspects go hand in hand.

The foundation of a great-looking physique is relative strength —a measure of how strong someone is in comparison to their own body weight. This is contrary to absolute strength, which measures the total force one can exert without considering body weight. Relative strength is important for aesthetics because it tells us about your muscle to fat ratio, i.e. higher relative strength means more muscle and less fat.

Training calisthenics naturally leads to lower body fat due to the mechanics of bodyweight exercise; the leaner you are, the better you become at moving your own weight. When you commit to calisthenics, every pound of fat shed directly translates to improved performance. This relationship creates a positive feedback loop between your diet and your exercise routine. Contrast this with weight training, where dropping body weight tends to decrease lifting performance. Decreased performance is frustrating and can often derail one's dietary efforts as they subconsciously try to maintain their lifting capabilities—this is why many people that lift weights find themselves stuck in the perpetual loop between cutting and bulking.

Calisthenics practitioners have great looking physiques precisely because they must stay lean. In this discipline, every pound gained needs to contribute to strength, not to excess fat. When lifting weights, gaining 20 pounds (half of it as fat) doesn't matter because you're lifting external weight rather than your body weight.

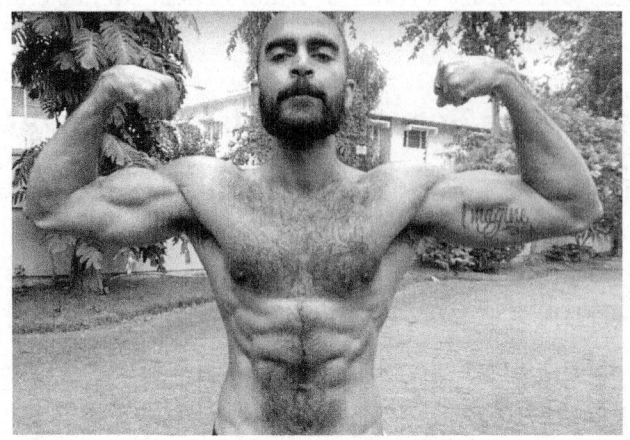

Bodyweight exercises naturally create a lean, muscular and defined physique.

The aesthetic appeal of a calisthenics practitioner is not just in their muscle definition but in the functional beauty their physique represents. It's not about the absolute strength of lifting as much weight as possible, but the relative strength of moving your own body with ease and grace. The result is a lean, defined, and functionally strong body – a true representation of health and fitness.

Accessibility: Your Body Is Your Gym

With calisthenics, your body is your gym and the world is your playground. You are liberated from the confines of a traditional gym, allowing you to engage in exercise wherever you are. You don't need to wait for your turn on the machine or commute to a fitness center. You can seamlessly integrate exercise into your daily routine – a set of push ups in your living room, squats in your office, or pull ups in a nearby park. This accessibility means less room for the usual 'no time' excuse.

Many of my private coaching clients travel for work. Staying consistent with workouts used to be a challenge for them but calisthenics came to the rescue, offering the flexibility to maintain a fitness routine from anywhere – even in a tiny hotel room.

One of the best things about calisthenics is being able to exercise outdoors. There's a unique charm in exercising under the open sky, feeling the warmth of the sun, and breathing in fresh air – a stark contrast to working out in the cramped and stuffy environment of a conventional gym. Outdoor exercise, be it in a park or on a beach, not only invigorates the body but also refreshes the mind.

The accessibility of calisthenics breaks down the barriers of equipment and location, inviting a freedom of practice that is as unbounded as it is practical. Whether in the comfort of your living room or in the expanse of a park, the ability to exercise is always at hand, unhindered by the need for elaborate equipment.

Proprioception: Awareness Through Space

A less discussed but very important benefit of bodyweight exercise is the improvement of proprioception — the body's intuitive sense of its position, motion, and equilibrium in space.

Calisthenics focuses on closed-chain exercises (like push ups, squats, chin ups etc.) where the hands or feet are fixed, as the body moves through space. This is in contrast to open-chain machine, dumbbell or barbell exercises (like leg press, bench press, bicep curls etc.) where the body remains stationary as the limbs move through space.

Closed-chain exercises naturally engage more muscle groups than open-chain exercises because they require total body stabilization. Aaron Alexander captures this point in his book, *The Align Method:*

> "Generally speaking, the more complex the fitness apparatus, the less intelligent the body needs to be in order to use it. Our brain is brilliant at conserving energy, and if you outsource the need to stabilize, balance, or use a range of motion to a machine, the muscles and neural connections innervated to perform those actions begin to atrophy and wither away."

For example, in order to perform reps on the leg press machine all that you require is the lower body strength to move a particular weight. To perform reps of full range of motion squats requires lower body strength and balance coupled with hip mobility, core stability and flexibility in the knees and ankles—all of these aspects are taken to the next level when performing squats on one leg instead of two. This emphasis on stability and muscle engagement is why closed-chain exercises are particularly effective in developing proprioception and kinesthetic awareness. As you progress in calisthenics, your body learns to navigate and adapt to various positions and movements, enhancing overall body awareness.

Confident, skillful movement starts with the basics, and through calisthenics, you'll discover how to systematically build your body's athletic foundation. This includes developing hip mobility, joint integrity, and coordination so you can move through space with elegance and grace. Feeling free in your own body to move the way you want is empowering. Motor control is a crucial aspect of this, and advancing with calisthenics gives you the confidence of knowing that your body is prepared to handle anything life throws at you.

Improved proprioception has far-reaching benefits, from better agility and reduced injury risk to enhanced performance in daily activities. As you master the art of propelling and stabilizing your own body weight, the communication between mind and muscle becomes more refined, enhancing your ability to navigate through space with precision.

Transferable Strength: Beyond The Bars

The results gained from calisthenics are not confined to the dimensions of a pull up bar or the limits of a routine. This style of exercise teaches your body to function as an integrated unit, harmonizing strength, balance, and coordination.

Consider the example of a push up. At first glance, it appears to be an exercise for the chest, shoulders and triceps. But performing reps with proper technique also requires many other muscle groups—including the lats, serratus anterior, abdominals, glutes, legs, tibialis and feet—to maintain an isometric contraction (meaning that these muscles must contract statically to stabilize the body). This total body engagement is what sets bodyweight exercise apart because it trains your muscle groups to work in unison rather than isolation. Such integration is fundamental to most sports and physical activities.

In soccer, for instance, a player needs the coordinated effort of their legs for running and kicking, their core for balance and direction change, and their upper body for power and stability. Activities in daily life also demand a combination of strength, balance, and coordination. Take the simple act of carrying a heavy box up a flight of stairs, for example. This task requires leg strength for climbing, core stability to maintain balance, and arm strength for holding the box. The integrated strength developed through calisthenics prepares the body for such real-life challenges, making these tasks feel less strenuous and reducing the risk of injury.

In essence, the strength gained from calisthenics is versatile and supports physical activity in general. The strength, agility, endurance, and total-body coordination developed spill over into everyday life, enhancing everything from recreational sports to the simple act of climbing stairs.

Beyond exercise, calisthenics is a holistic discipline that molds the body, sharpens the mind, and enhances overall well-being. It is an ancient path redefined by modern understanding, one that we will continue to explore and celebrate in the pages to come.

The Warrior Essence: Strength Through Adaptation

In the heart of ancient Sparta, there lived a warrior named Leonidas.

Leonidas' story is one of a soldier whose physique was built not in lavish gyms but upon the unforgiving terrain of his homeland. His muscles were carved through the mastery of moving his own body weight, giving rise to a form that was lean, efficient, and versatile. This natural adaptation not only contributed to an imposing appearance but also ensured his readiness for the unpredictable demands of battle.

The tales of his exploits speak not of a man who sought fitness but one who lived it. His training was his life; his body was his gym. In the minimalist spirit of Spartan tradition, Leonidas found freedom. He didn't require elaborate equipment and was therefore able to maintain his peak condition whether at home or on the move.

In combat, Leonidas' strength was as much about the keen awareness of his body in space as it was about physical power. It was this integrated approach that fortified him against injury and gave his movements a grace and fluidity that seemed almost supernatural.

The legend of Leonidas teaches us a timeless truth:

The essence of calisthenics is not merely in the accumulation of individual benefits but in the holistic elevation of the human form and function.

Leonidas' legacy is a testament to the power of adaptability and the impact of a training philosophy that is simple, yet profoundly effective — a philosophy that shapes not only how one looks but how one lives and thrives in the face of challenges.

Cultivating Full-Body Functionality

In this chapter, we've ventured through the practical and transformative world of calisthenics, uncovering the many benefits it offers.

We've learned about supple strength and how bodyweight exercise naturally leans you out, prevents injury, is convenient, improves proprioception, builds aesthetic muscle, and develops transferable functional strength.

Remember, calisthenics is not a fitness fad; it's a return to our roots, providing a foundation for a sustainable, strong, and capable body.

As we leave behind the advantages of calisthenics, it's essential to approach our journey with eyes wide open. The road to peak physical adaptability is not without its challenges.

In the spirit of complete transparency and to give you a well-rounded perspective, our next chapter confronts the often glossed-over aspects of bodyweight exercise. Here, we will expose the limitations that accompany this ancient yet ever-relevant form of physical training.

The upcoming chapter doesn't take away from the value

of calisthenics but rather provides a candid, full-spectrum view. An honest approach ensures that you, the reader, are empowered to make informed decisions, acknowledging not only where calisthenics excels but also where it may fall short.

Join me as we dive into the disadvantages of bodyweight exercise, ensuring that our fitness philosophy is not only founded on adaptability and strength but also on the wisdom that comes from recognizing and working with our limitations.

Chapter Takeaways

- Calisthenics builds supple strength, combining strength and flexibility, crucial for explosive movements and injury prevention.

- Transitioning to calisthenics can reduce and even heal chronic injuries, as these exercises promote proper body alignment and balance muscle with connective tissue development.

- Achieving a lean, muscular physique is a natural result of bodyweight exercise because the leaner you are, the easier it is to lift your body weight against gravity.

- Calisthenics can be performed anywhere, anytime, breaking the limitations of traditional gym environments and equipment.

- Calisthenics improve proprioception, enhancing the body's spatial awareness and coordination.

- The strength gained from bodyweight exercises is versatile and applicable to a variety of physical activities and daily tasks.

- Calisthenics embodies the principles of adaptability and holistic fitness, echoing the ancient wisdom of training for functionality and resilience.

CHAPTER 3 - CALISTHENICS DOWNSIDES

"I never allow myself to hold an opinion on anything that I don't know the other side's argument better than they do."

—CHARLIE MUNGER

The doctor's words were a cold splash of reality, "Surgery is the best option," he said, examining the scans that displayed torn cartilage in my right knee. I sat there, digesting the possibility of the knife, the anesthesia, and the long road to recovery. It was a crossroads moment, the kind where life seems to lean in and whisper, "Is this really the best option?"

I had always chased the image of strength—the broad shoulders, the sculpted arms, the square pecs I could show off at the beach. Frankly, I enjoyed the glances I got from strangers. But I hid the price of that enjoyment. My neglected lower body, the very basis of my physique, was weak and underdeveloped, a secret I guarded as fiercely as I pursued my 'beach muscles.'

I had skipped training legs not once but routinely. The imbalance was not just in my physique but in my approach. And it cost me—first my right knee, then my left, each tear of cartilage was a harsh lesson in the price of vanity.

As I weighed my options, surgery or not, I reflected on my journey—how shame at the swimming pool led me to lifting weights at the gym. Now, I was sitting at the doctor's office with broad shoulders, big arms, square pecs and torn knees.

Eventually, it was the path of calisthenics that began to heal my legs, not through scalpel and stitches, but through the very balance I had once ignored. Yet, even as my knees found relief, my legs remained a step behind in development—pointing to the glaring downside of bodyweight exercise. It's the untold story of the difficulty in developing legs to match the upper body when the weight you lift is limited to your own.

This story isn't just a tale of personal oversight but a prelude to the challenge we face with calisthenics. It's a challenge that speaks to the very core of our physical pursuits—balance, proportion, and the symmetry of strength.

So I chose the road less scalpelled, but not without its own set of sharp truths. And as I share this, I invite you to explore the nuanced reality of calisthenics. Let's dive into the disadvantages of exercising with bodyweight, starting with the admission that not all muscles are made equal in the gravity-bound gym of your own flesh and bones.

Disadvantages Of Bodyweight Exercise

In the realm of fitness, every discipline carries its weight in gold and its weight in shadows. Calisthenics is no exception.

The advantages of exercising with bodyweight are numerous

and compelling as discussed in the previous chapter. Yet, there is also a counter-narrative—a story less told but equally instructive. The disadvantages of bodyweight exercise, while not diminishing its value, add crucial brushstrokes to the complete picture of this practice. In this chapter, we will explore these lesser-spoken truths with an honest lens. We will dive into the challenges of developing certain muscle groups, the complexities of scaling difficulty, and the realities that arise when the only weight you lift is your own.

Understanding the drawbacks of calisthenics is not an exercise in discouragement, but rather, it's about setting realistic expectations. My aim with this book is to arm you with knowledge—both of what bodyweight exercise can generously offer and what it may, at times, withhold. Let's begin with the most fundamental aspect—the challenge of developing substantial lower body mass.

The Limitation Of Size And Strength In The Lower Body

The lower body contains some of the largest and most powerful muscles in the human body—glutes, quads, calves and hamstrings. While bodyweight exercises can develop these muscles to be strong and functional, they often fall short in building the sheer size and power achievable through weightlifting.

Bodyweight exercises typically develop muscle that is more athletic rather than large. This is not to understate the effectiveness of calisthenics; exercises like single-leg squats can build remarkable strength in the lower-body. Yet, in my personal journey and experimentation, I've attempted sets of barbell squats after I started calisthenics and it's obvious that the strength in my lower body, developed through single-leg squats, lags behind the more advanced capabilities of my upper body.

Bodyweight exercises can build strong, capable legs but not necessarily the larger, hypertrophied muscles that can only come through heavy weightlifting.

Athletic Vs. Aesthetic Perspective

A common debate I encounter is the effectiveness of bodyweight exercise for certain fitness goals. Some argue that calisthenics is not suitable for every aspiration and this is partly true. Let's start by distinguishing between the two fitness objectives of athletic ability and aesthetic appearance.

If your aim is to enhance functional fitness – the kind of strength and agility useful in sports and everyday life – calisthenics shines. On the other hand, if your goal is to step on stage as a bodybuilder or compete in a powerlifting competition, then calisthenics falls short. The arena of bodybuilding requires a specific, bulky muscle aesthetic while powerlifting requires the ability to lift extremely heavy external weights. In such cases, bodyweight exercises shouldn't be your main focus because they are less effective at building the kind of large muscle size and sheer strength necessary for these pursuits.

I know this point may seem obvious, but it's worth mentioning because people debate me on this all the time—even though I agree with them. Calisthenics is great for building a functionally fit and athletic physique. But if your aim is to enter a bodybuilding or powerlifting competition, then lifting weights is essential. Understanding this distinction helps in aligning your training method with your fitness goals, whether they are athletic, aesthetic or both.

The Challenge Of Progressive Overload

Progressive overload is the practice of continuously increasing exercise intensity as your body gets stronger. With weightlifting, progressive overload is a simple matter of adding more weight to the bar, using heavier dumbbells, or increasing the resistance level on a machine. With calisthenics, progressive overload is more complex because the weight you lift is your own. And though it's possible to exert a tremendous amount of resistance on the upper body without external weights, this is not the case with the lower body. Beyond a certain point, your legs need more resistance than your body weight can provide in order to grow larger.

With weightlifting, incrementally adding weight to the bar is a clear and quantifiable method of progression. With calisthenics, increasing exercise intensity to stimulate muscle growth requires more creativity and is less measurable.

Rate Of Muscle Growth

Packing on muscle mass with bodyweight exercise is a slower process when compared to weightlifting because factors like balance, mobility, and joint stability play a role in proper exercise execution. These factors, while contributing to full-body functionality, can also limit muscle gains. For instance, let's say that your lower-body has more than enough strength to perform a single-leg squat. But if your balance, mobility, stability and/or coordination are lacking, then you will be unable to fully express your strength on this exercise leading to less muscle gains. On the other hand, if you're on the leg press machine, then you can lift near your true strength potential because factors like balance, stability or mobility aren't limiting factors.

Also remember from our discussion in the previous chapter that muscle tissue adapts to resistance at a much faster rate than connective tissue due to its higher blood flow, which aids in recovery and growth. Advanced bodyweight exercises require a high level of connective tissue strength but this is not necessarily the case with weightlifting. For example, working up to single-arm push ups requires strong hands, wrists and elbows. But you can work up to a very heavy weight on the chest press machine without placing any stress on your wrists or elbows.

Those aiming to pack on as much muscle and strength as possible in the shortest amount of time may find calisthenics to be a supplement rather than the prime focus of their workout routine.

The Lesson Of Function Over Form

It was the peak of summer, and I remember the sun casting long shadows on the pavement as I walked down the street. My pace quickened with a sense of discomfort. My legs, particularly my calves, felt overly exposed in the shorts I was reluctantly wearing. They were, in my eyes, pencil thin—far from the robust pillars I envisioned as a hallmark of strength. I avoided wearing shorts on most days, haunted by an insecurity that had become part of my self-perception.

No matter the reps, the sets, and the aching burn from single-leg squats and calf raises, my lower body refused to grow like my upper body. My legs and calves remained underdeveloped and resistant to my efforts.

The obsession for getting huge legs took a turn one evening as I stumbled upon highlights from a UFC fight. My fascination with combat sports had grown as I started training martial arts myself. On the screen, Jon Jones—a name synonymous with dominance in the sport of Mixed martial arts (MMA)—moved with a predatory grace, his calves lean, almost invisible. Yet, there he was, an embodiment of combat efficiency.

I remember leaning forward, my eyes tracing the fighters' movements, a realization slowly dawning on me. Jon Jones, despite his thinner legs, was dominating opponents with a precise blend of technique and functional power. His body was a finely tuned instrument of athleticism, not an ornament of muscle mass. It was a contrast to the heavy-legged musculature I had been admiring on bodybuilders.

Over time, as I engaged more deeply with martial arts, the truth became self-evident. The functionality of my body—the power in my punches, the strength of my grappling, the whip in my kicks, and the conditioning of my cardio—had all improved, not in spite of my calisthenics training, but because of it. My joints remained sturdy, unburdened by excessive weight yet fortified by consistent, varied movement.

This was my moment of clarity:

Functionality is the true currency in the economy of physicality, not the size of one's calves or the bulk of one's thighs.

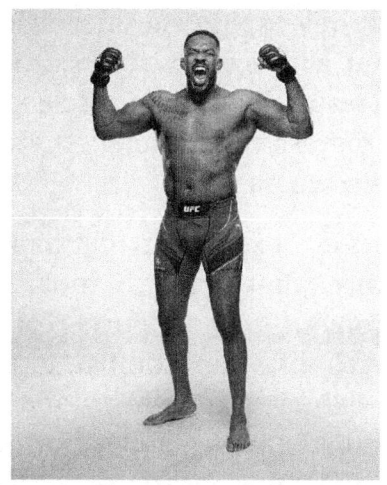

Arguably the most dominant fighter to ever grace the sport of Mixed martial arts, Jon Jones, had pencil thin-calves and tiny quads even as a heavyweight.

The mirror had lied; cage fighting spoke the truth. Calisthenics had not sculpted me into a musclebound hunk, but it had forged me into something perhaps more vital—a functional athlete, equipped for the comprehensive demands of Mixed martial arts, the ultimate physical chess.

The story of my pencil thin calves, once a source of shame, became a narrative of empowerment, teaching me that the aesthetics of muscle could never trump the superior utility of functional strength. This epiphany, born from the juxtaposition of my own insecurities and the excellence of a champion fighter, crystallized the essence of what calisthenics offered—pure functionality, a truth as evident in combat as it was in life's daily battles.

Strength Beyond Size

As we close this chapter, remember the core lesson:

Calisthenics is not a fast track to muscle gains, but it is a path to functional, athletic strength.

While it's true that developing significant lower body mass is challenging without additional weights, and that bodyweight exercise will not result in rapid muscle gains or allow for straightforward progressive overload, the true value of this training style lies elsewhere.

Bodyweight exercise excels in enhancing full body-coordination, balance, joint strength, mobility, and stability. It is about the functionality that supports real-world movements and activities—much like the combat effectiveness seen in elite fighters who exhibit strength beyond mere muscle size. Understand that calisthenics is about optimizing your body's natural abilities, not just its appearance.

In the opening of this chapter, I shared with you a personal crossroad—the doctor's suggestion of surgery for my knee and my decision to choose a different path. It was a moment that highlighted a crucial fact: our bodies are built for function, not just form. Reflect on Jon Jones, a champion whose thin calves disguise his functional power. My journey, like his, highlights that the essence of true strength is not always visible to the eye.

As we turn the page from theory to practice, we shift fc towards implementation. The upcoming chapters are abou laying the groundwork for your journey—a foundation upon which functional strength, athletic performance, and perhaps most importantly, personal well-being can be built.

We will explore the multiple dimensions of fitness, uncover the mathematics of aesthetics, and dive into the laws of lifting. Get ready to build upon what you've learned, to solidify your knowledge, and to take the next step in sculpting not just a body, but a capable, resilient, and functional form that's ready for the diverse challenges life throws at you.

With each chapter, we're not just training muscles; we're cultivating a mindset, a lifestyle, and a philosophy of strength that goes beyond the superficial, reaching for something more enduring and profound.

Chapter Takeaways

- Calisthenics, while effective for creating lean, functional legs, falls short in building the sheer lower-body size and strength achievable through weightlifting.

- Bodyweight exercises are great for functional fitness and athletic performance, but less suitable if you're aiming to compete as a bodybuilder or powerlifter.

- Calisthenics lacks the straightforward progressive overload of weightlifting, making it more challenging to continuously increase workout intensity.

- Muscle development with calisthenics training is slower compared to weightlifting, due to the requirement of factors like balance, joint strength, and stability.

CHAPTER 4 - THE TOTAL FITNESS PYRAMID

"Humans are not physically normal in the absence of hard physical effort. Exercise is not a thing we do to fix a problem – it is a thing we must do anyway, a thing without which there will always be problems."

—MARK RIPPETOE

What is exercise?

At first glance, this question seems simplistic, almost rhetorical. But as someone who understands that words are not just symbols but powerful tools shaping our perceptions, I invite you to join me in a brief, yet profound exploration.

As per the New Oxford American Dictionary, exercise is defined as *'activity requiring physical effort, carried on to sustain or improve health and fitness.'* But let's dive deeper, borrowing from the clarity that etymology provides. The Latin origins of the word *'exercise'* join *'ex-'*, meaning *'thoroughly'*, with *'arcere'*, meaning to *'contain'* or *'enclose'*. When combined, we arrive at *'exercere'*, meaning to *'keep at work'*. The roots of this word suggest a continuous engagement, a persistent effort to harness the body's vitality. The Late Latin *'exercitium'* further evolves this into *'training'*, adding a dimension of purpose and progression.

In the modern world, many have lost touch with the importance of exercise. It is seen as optional, rather than an essential part of daily life. We witness the consequences in our communities where vitality and physical capacity are diminishing from lack of use. This detachment from our intrinsic need for movement not only encloses us within physical limitations but often within mental ones as well.

Reflecting on the Latin etymology, exercise isn't just about movement—it's about sustenance. Exercise is a means to thoroughly contain and cultivate the body's energies and abilities. And it's within this context that we will consider exercise not as a task or chore but as a vital practice to nurture and expand our physical horizons.

Let us then redefine exercise, not as a mere act of physical labor but as any activity that keeps our bodies at work so that they grow in capability; activities that contain the life force within so that vigor and health is not lost. With this definition in mind, we can construct a pyramid of fitness, laying each stone with purpose, aiming not just to build strength, stamina, or muscle but to reclaim the essence of our well-being.

As we step into this chapter, keep in mind that true exercise is an art—carefully crafted, consistently practiced, and deeply understood. It's an art that weaves strength into our limbs and breathes capacity into our lungs. It is, indeed, the work of keeping our very essence enclosed within a fortress of health and vitality.

A Framework For Full-Body Functionality

We're about to unfold a framework for holistic physical fitness. I will guide you through the multiple aspects of fitness so that you can begin to view it as a rich spectrum of capabilities rather than a one-dimensional attribute. From the raw strength required to lift and the endurance necessary for a marathon, to the grace of a dancer and the balance in a steady stance—each is a crucial piece of the puzzle.

TOTAL FITNESS BLUEPRINT

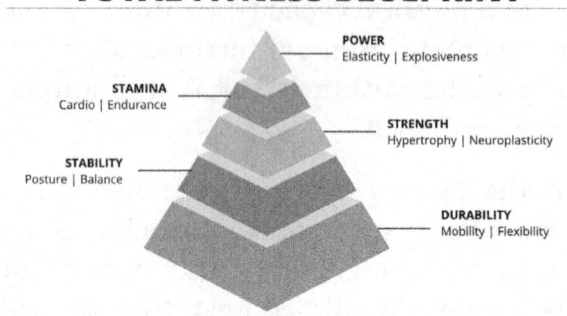

- **POWER** — Elasticity | Explosiveness
- **STAMINA** — Cardio | Endurance
- **STRENGTH** — Hypertrophy | Neuroplasticity
- **STABILITY** — Posture | Balance
- **DURABILITY** — Mobility | Flexibility

Developing full-body fitness and functionality means developing the multiple dimensions of fitness including durability, stability, strength, stamina and power.

Imagine your body as a vessel of untapped potential. To experience its vast capabilities, we must go beyond conventional workouts. We must craft a routine that cultivates our movement abilities so that we can enjoy and excel in the activities that enrich our lives.

By the end of this chapter, you'll have a clear understanding of how to build a foundation that is both strong and versatile. You'll learn how to develop a fitness routine that respects the complexity of your body's needs, creating balance and harmony in your physical form.

Prepare to challenge what you know about fitness, to push the boundaries of your abilities, and to redefine what your body can achieve. This is the essence of our exploration—the construction of a body temple that stands strong and adaptable in the face of life's demands.

Let's dive in.

Layer #1 - Durability: Joint Fluidity

At the base of our pyramid lies durability—a term that's linked to mobility and flexibility. Building a durable physique means building your body from the ground up, ensuring every joint, from your toes to your neck, can handle stress and move fluidly.

Joints are formed where two or more bones meet and they serve as the pivot points on which your body's movement and stability depend. They can vary in structure and function, but they generally contain several important elements that work together to enable motion, absorb shock, and protect the bones from wear and tear. Within a joint are various connective tissues like tendons, ligaments, and cartilage. Unlike muscles, which can quickly receive oxygen and nutrients through increased blood flow during exercise, connective tissues rely on compression, tension, and movement of the joints to pump synovial fluid into the areas around the cartilage and ligaments. This fluidity is essential for maintaining joint function and also contributes to mobility and flexibility. People often use these terms interchangeably, but mobility and flexibility are two different aspects of physicality.

Flexibility is the ability of your muscles to stretch and lengthen. It's about how far you can enter into a range of motion when an external force (like your arms or gravity) is helping you. For example, when you reach down to touch your toes, how far you can go depends on the flexibility of your hamstrings.

Mobility is the ability of your joints to move through a particular range of motion with control. It's not just about how far you can move, but how well you can move actively and with strength. For example, if you can squat down all the way to where your hamstrings touch your calves, and then stand back up smoothly, that's an example of mobility. It shows that your knees, hips, and ankles can move through that range of motion while supporting your body weight.

Simply put, flexibility is passive—it's about how far your muscles can stretch. Mobility is active—it's about how well your joints can move through their range of motion with strength and control. In other words, flexibility is about how much your muscles can lengthen, while mobility is about how well you can use that length to move your joints effectively. Both are important for overall physical fitness, but they serve different purposes. You can be flexible (able to touch your toes), but if you can't control your movement (like squatting deeply with control), you might still have poor mobility.

> *"Flexibility allows you to bend, not break, under the pressures of life and the stressors of a workout. Mobility allows you to complete wider ranges of motion without unnecessary compensation or additional pain."*
>
> **–Aubrey Marcus**

In my exploration of various fitness disciplines, gymnastics is what taught me the importance of joint mobility. Gymnasts prioritize joint mobilization because they routinely perform exercises that place significant stress on their joints. Advanced gymnastics exercises are beyond the scope of this book, but in an upcoming chapter you will discover a series of exercises to mobilize every major joint in your body. Mobility training means taking care of the connective tissues and intricate structures within your joints to ensure they stay lubricated and capable of taking on load. This style of training shields you against potential injuries and also improves overall strength training performance.

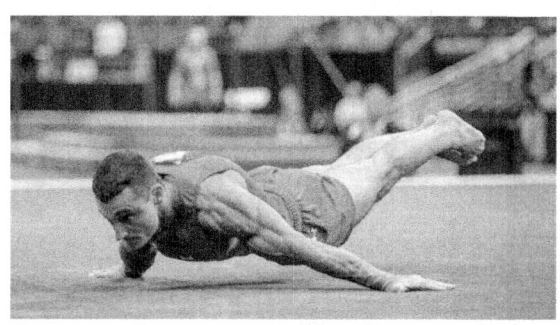

The Maltese, as demonstrated by elite gymnast Brandon Wynn, places a tremendous amount of strain on the wrists, elbows, shoulders and entire spine. Gymnasts prioritize joint mobility because their sport demands it.

Flexibility is the second component of maintaining a durable physique. Life inevitably places us in vulnerable positions, whether it's twisting an ankle on a hike, reaching beyond our normal range to pick something up off the floor, or getting caught in a submission attempt while training Brazilian jiu-jitsu. Being flexible can protect against injury in these situations. Flexibility is not just about achieving extreme ranges of motion for the sake of it; it's about ensuring that your body can handle unexpected demands without experiencing harm.

Durability is the base upon which all other dimensions of fitness rest. By ensuring mobile joints and flexible muscles, you're setting the stage for a balanced, injury-free, and holistic approach to fitness, one that truly embodies the ethos of being fit for life.

A study on the Sitting-Rising Test (SRT) published in the European Journal of Preventive Cardiology reveals the practical importance of constructing a durable foundation for longevity. The SRT involves a straightforward task — sitting down on the floor and then standing back up, with the scoring based on the amount of support needed. A total of 10 points are possible, with points deducted for each support used, like a hand or knee. The study uncovered a striking correlation between SRT scores and mortality. It found that individuals requiring more support (and thus scoring lower) to sit and rise from the floor had a higher rate of mortality. Specifically, each point decrease in the test was linked to a 21% increase in death from all causes[1].

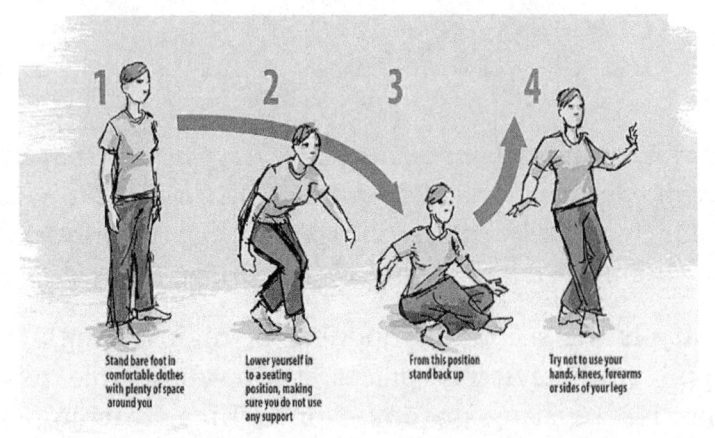

The SRT reflects the mobility and flexibility of the ankles, knees, hips, glutes, hamstrings, calves, and back.

The ease with which one can move, sit, and rise is not just a matter of convenience or athletic ability; it is a marker of how well our bodies can sustain and support us through the years. Therefore, the more you condition your joints to be mobile and your muscles to be flexible, the more durable and capable your body becomes.

Layer #2 - Stability: Core Integrity

As we ascend to the next layer of our pyramid, we arrive at stability. Specifically, we're speaking of core stability and its impact on posture and balance. Building a strong and stable core is often misunderstood as the pursuit of toned abdominals. But your core is actually the entire area that wraps around your torso - a central link in the kinetic chain that keeps your body centered and balanced. It includes the muscles of your abdomen, lower back, hips, and even your diaphragm.

Our aim is to have a core that is functional — one that supports your body in everyday movements and athletic pursuits alike. Part of building full-body fitness means that your body's strength is anchored by a stable core.

The stability of your core directly influences your posture because it supports the spine in maintaining proper alignment. Proper posture projects confidence, yes, and it also prevents chronic conditions like thoracic kyphosis (hunchback) and lumbar lordosis (swayback). Building a stable core is crucial for avoiding long-term spinal issues. The core also helps distribute weight and manage physical stresses, preventing common issues like lower back pain.

Moreover, core stability is essential for balance and agility. Whether in sporting activities or daily chores, your core is what allows you to move with greater control and efficiency. It is this balance, stemming from a stable core, that helps prevent falls — a leading cause of injury, particularly as we age[2].

Core stability is the bridge that connects muscular development to functional capability. A weak core cannot control excessive movement, creating energy leaks and reduced efficiency. In contrast, a strong and stable core ensures proper force distribution during heavy and explosive movements, safeguarding the spine.

In striking martial arts, the principle is clear: the stronger your core, the more effectively you can channel energy from the ground through your lower body, up to your extremities. Your core links the rotation of your hips to your upper back, essential for powerful punches. Practically all major sporting movements that involve the feet being planted on the ground – like sprinting, jumping, twisting, throwing, and cutting – engage the core extensively. But having a strong and stable core goes beyond athletic performance; it's about quality of life.

Calisthenics demands immense core activation, especially as you progress towards advanced exercises like dips and pull ups, because a stable core is essential for maintaining your body's balance during these movements. With bodyweight exercises, developing superior core strength and coordination is non-negotiable. Remarkably, you can achieve perfectly developed six pack abs without the need for direct abdominal work, making your training both efficient and effective.

In the grand scheme of longevity, core stability is a cornerstone. It's about preventing falls, maintaining posture, and ensuring that our bodies can support us through the varied challenges of life. A stable core is synonymous with a body that can adapt, endure, and thrive — the very essence of living a long and healthy life.

With calisthenics, every push, pull, squat, and hold is a step towards sculpting a core that is strong, stable, functional and enduring. As we embrace stability, we embrace a life of balance, strength, and vitality.

Layer #3 - Strength: Muscular Force

Next, we encounter the vital layer of strength that can be broken down into the two components of muscular hypertrophy, or muscle size, and neuromuscular efficiency, or the quality of muscle contractions.

The relationship between your nervous system and muscular system can be compared to the relationship between an electrical circuit and a light bulb. Think of your nervous system as the circuitry and your muscles as the light bulb. Just as increasing the wattage of an electrical circuit makes a bulb glow brighter, enhancing neuromuscular efficiency – through improved motor unit recruitment – makes your muscles contract harder, allowing for more strength.

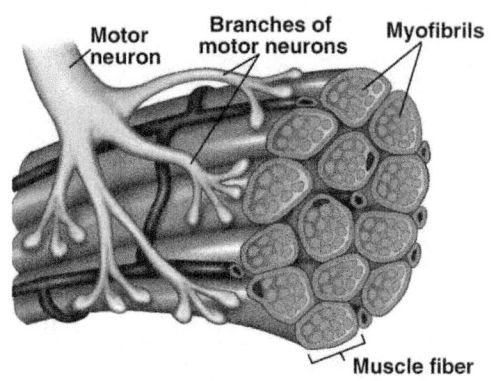

Muscular contractions are triggered by signals from the nervous system, with motor neurons activating muscle fibers through their branches, allowing coordinated movement and strength.

Bodybuilders focus on increasing muscle size, which in our analogy translates to building a bigger light bulb. But no matter how big a lightbulb is in size, the amount of light it gives off depends on the amount of wattage coming through the circuit. A trained fighter may look skinny, but he is able to throw harder punches and kicks than a bulky bodybuilder because he's able to bring more 'wattage' into his muscles by recruiting muscle fibers more efficiently.

Ultimately, whether through muscle growth or neuromuscular efficiency, our goal is to increase the 'light' – which in this context means more strength or greater work output from the muscles. The key is in understanding how to utilize both components of strength effectively.

Tying back to our overarching goal of longevity, research indicates higher muscular strength to be linked to a lower risk of death from any cause and specifically from cancer[3]. In fact, men with the lowest muscular strength had a 50% higher rate of death from all causes compared to those in the middle third of muscular strength[4]. This underscores the importance of strength not just for immediate physical capabilities but also for our overarching goal of living a long and healthy life.

Layer #4 - Stamina: Sustained Effort

Ascending further up the pyramid, we encounter stamina, the fuel that powers your ability to maintain effort over time, whether in a long-distance run, a rigorous hike, or a circuit training workout.

Stamina is composed of two elements. The first is aerobic capacity, which is your cardiovascular fitness, and the second is muscular endurance. The difference between cardio and endurance depends on whether it is your aerobic capacity (your lungs) or muscular fatigue that limits your ability to sustain physical effort. For example, jogging for as long as you can would be a test of your aerobic capacity or cardio. But holding a plank for as long as you can would be a test of your muscular endurance. Both are critical components of stamina, each playing a unique role in overall fitness.

Your aerobic capacity, measured as VO_2 max (maximum oxygen uptake), is based on how efficiently your body can deliver and utilize oxygen to produce energy in your muscles. VO_2 max is a measure of cardiovascular fitness, determining your body's ability to support sustained physical activity.

Like all layers of the pyramid, our pursuit of stamina also impacts our goal of longevity. Studies have found low aerobic capacity in middle-aged men to be associated with increased mortality rates. Each increase in VO_2 max levels is linked with a 21% lower risk of death over 45 years of follow up even after adjusting for risk factors such as smoking, blood pressure and cholesterol[5]. However, it's vital to recognize the point of diminishing returns. Long distance runners, for example, may have high VO_2 max but they also have high injury rates[6] which highlights the need for a balanced approach to cardio. Other studies show that excessively running long-distances can lead to patchy myocardial fibrosis[7] (scarring on the heart's muscle tissue).

Jim Fixx, author of *The Complete Book of Running,* played a significant role in popularizing running as a form of exercise in the 70s. While his contribution to getting people active is commendable, his story also serves as a cautionary tale. Fixx died of a heart attack at the age of 52 while jogging. His story is a reminder of the importance of moderation and balance in our fitness approach.

Our focus is on building stamina that enhances fitness without compromising health. We'll explore routines and exercises that boost both your aerobic capacity and muscular endurance, ensuring they contribute positively to your long-term health and fitness goals.

Layer #5 - Power: Speed Of Force

Power crowns our pyramid by combining its two dynamic components of elasticity and explosiveness. Elasticity is your muscles' ability to snap back after being stretched (think of the recoil in a boxer's punch). Explosiveness is the ability to generate rapid force (like the burst of a sprinter at the starting gun).

If strength is the force that acts against resistance to create movement, then power is the rate at which that force is generated—it's about strength expressed with speed. Power is particularly important for competitive athletes because it directly impacts performance in activities requiring rapid, intense movements. Many high-level athletic training systems prioritize power development because it dictates how hard you can throw a punch, how explosively you can jump, or how fast you can throw a ball. In essence, developing physical power is about maximizing force generation.

Power is important, but it's also the most taxing on the body. For sports enthusiasts or those engaging in everyday fitness, intensive power training is not a necessity. The goal is to develop enough power when needed – whether it's sprinting or jumping away from danger, or defending yourself when necessary – without overtaxing the nervous system.

Training for power involves dynamic movements, including elements of plyometrics. Exercises like sprinting are also excellent for developing power. However, as noted earlier, for those not engaged in competitive athletics, developing this aspect of fitness doesn't need to be a priority.

From Overwhelm To Balance

There was a time when I thought 'getting fit' meant gaining muscle and losing fat. This was before my knee injuries.

The second tear of my left knee was more than an injury; it was a clear message that I was on the wrong path. The imbalance in my body was a reflection of an imbalance in my approach to fitness. I'd been pushing hard, but not smart.

Adversity often leads to insight, and in the quiet of recovery, I dove deep into the study of health, fitness, and exercise. I found that fitness was a multifaceted gem—strength, yes, but also joint mobility, core stability, cardio, stamina and power.

Eager for transformation, I constructed a routine as varied as it was intense: yoga twice a week for durability, strength training thrice a week to build strength and muscle, challenging hikes on the weekends to develop cardio and muscular endurance, dedicated stretching sessions in the evenings to get flexible and plyometric drills from time to time for explosiveness.

In my quest for peak physical condition, I had missed birthday parties, family dinners and evenings with friends—moments that life's memories are made of. Fitness was no longer enhancing my life; it was consuming it. That realization hit me hard.

Was there not a middle path? A way to cultivate complete fitness without losing the essence of living?

These questions set me on a new quest—not for more, but for enough. The 'minimum effective dose' of exercise that would allow me to build a body capable of enjoying life's adventures without becoming the sole adventure itself. In a later chapter, we'll construct a refined, singular routine that develops the multiple aspects of fitness without taking over your life.

To wrap up this chapter, realize that fitness is an expansive concept, built on a foundation that is as diverse as it is integral. We started with the understanding that to exercise is to thoroughly engage our body's capacities. Then we went layer by layer through the 'Fitness Pyramid'—beginning with the base of durability and ascending through core stability, strength, stamina, and power. Remember, while the layers of the pyramid are distinct, they are not separate. Each aspect supports and enhances the others, contributing to a holistic approach to health, fitness, and longevity.

As we loop back to our opening discussion on the roots of 'exercise', recall the essence of keeping our body's energies and capacities actively contained. Each facet of fitness serves this purpose, ensuring that our physical form is not just a vessel, but a vibrant, capable, and resilient expression of life.

As we turn the page from understanding the breadth of fitness to the quest for aesthetic harmony, we'll explore how the ancient Greeks not only sought strength and functionality but also an ideal of beauty in human form. They perceived the human body as a canvas for sculptural art, guided by mathematical principles that created symmetry and proportion. The next chapter will deconstruct these timeless aesthetics, revealing how they are not relics of a past era but relevant markers for our fitness journey today. We will unlock the secrets of proportion that can transform the body into a living sculpture, mirroring the classical ideals that continue to inspire in the realm of physical excellence.

Join me as we shift our focus from the robust fitness pyramid to the artistry of its expression—where fitness meets form, function meets beauty, and where every physical endeavor is an act of creation in the pursuit of your personal masterpiece.

Chapter Takeaways

- Fitness is a multidimensional attribute that goes beyond just building muscle and losing fat. It encompasses a range of capabilities including joint mobility, flexibility, core stability, stamina, strength, and power, all contributing to overall well-being.

- Fluid joints are the base of your fitness and well-being, crucial for injury prevention and overall body resilience.

- A strong and stable core is vital not just for athletic performance but for daily activities and safety. The core is about more than just your abs; it encompasses the entire torso and is your body's center of gravity.

- Strength is not just about muscle size (hypertrophy). It is also about neuromuscular efficiency which is how efficiently your brain sends signals to your muscles and how effectively your muscles respond to those signals to produce force and movement.

- Stamina, combining aerobic capacity and muscular endurance, is crucial for long-term health. It's important to balance stamina training with other fitness aspects to avoid overtraining and injuries.

- Power combines elasticity and explosiveness, essential for high-level athletic performance. For non-athletes, sufficient power is necessary for everyday activities requiring quick, strong movements.

Success Check-In Exercise

Before moving on, let's gauge where you're at in the different dimensions of fitness.

This subjective assessment is helpful for two reasons:

1. It will help clarify how you evaluate yourself in the different aspects of fitness.
2. It will help set a reference point for yourself, so you can evaluate which areas need the most focus.

Don't think too much, use the first number that comes up in your head and heart.

Rate how true these statements are to you on a scale from 1 to 10.
(1 - least true; 10 - most true)

Rate how true these statements are to you on a scale from 1 to 10. (1 - least true; 10 - most true)	Your rating
Joint health: My body is free from injury and moves freely without pain.	
Flexibility: My body is flexible without much tightness or stiffness.	
Muscle mass and strength: I am very happy with my body's strength level and muscle composition.	
Aesthetics: I am very satisfied with how my body looks.	
Stamina: I can keep a high level of physical	

activity without getting tired.	
Power: I can easily jump, sprint and lift heavy objects fast and safely.	
Feel: My body moves and feels as if I'm in the best shape of my life.	
Performance: I feel like my body is primed and optimized to keep high performance for many years to come.	
Total fitness: I am very happy with my overall level of fitness.	

CHAPTER 5 - SCULPTING SYMMETRY

"Perfection comes about little by little through many numbers."

—POLYKLEITOS

Muscles tensed, a man stands in the grand hall of a museum, his eyes focused on the ancient statues before him. This is no ordinary visitor; this is Eugen Sandow, a man destined to become the father of modern bodybuilding. His gaze is not of simple admiration but of a calculated study, a quest to unlock the secret of perfect human proportions.

As visitors pass by, unaware, Sandow moves with purpose, tape measure in hand. He measures the arms, legs, and torsos of ancient sculptures that have stood the test of time. This is his laboratory with the marble and bronze statues as his subjects. Sandow is uncovering a code, an ancient code of physical excellence that he would come to call 'The Grecian Ideal'.

Unlike modern bodybuilders who focus exclusively on maximizing muscle mass, Sandow sought a balance of form and strength. His quest was not merely to grow in size but to sculpt his body into a living example of classical beauty and athletic ability. He carefully noted his findings, turning these measurements into a blueprint for his own transformation.

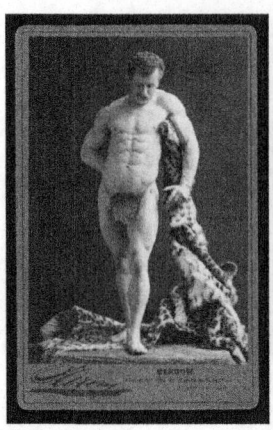

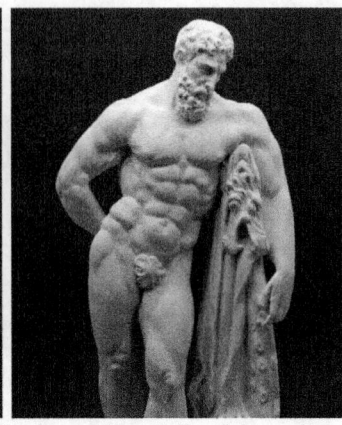

Sandow is known as the father of bodybuilding (in fact, he may have even coined the term) because he was the first person in recorded history to consciously sculpt his physique according to predetermined measurements.

In his books, *Strength and How to Obtain It* and *Sandow's System of Physical Training*, Sandow shares a philosophy of symmetry and proportion. His teachings focus on sculpting a physique that harmonizes with a divine proportion that mathematicians call the Golden Ratio.

In this chapter, we will uncover the principles of the Golden Ratio and how they can be applied to achieve a body that is strong, athletic and aesthetically balanced. You'll discover how Sandow's legacy extends beyond fitness, into the realms of art and beauty, and how you can apply his timeless principles to sculpt your own body into a work of living art.

The Theory Of Ideal Proportions

In our exploration of aesthetics, we're not just talking about muscle proportions; we're uncovering a fascinating intersection between art, science, and history. This journey begins with Euclid, an ancient Greek mathematician, who first defined the Golden Ratio in his seminal work, *Elements*. His definition laid the foundation for understanding this mysterious number that subtly guides the sacred geometry of our universe.

Two quantities have the Golden Ratio when their sum divided by the larger quantity equals the larger quantity divided by the smaller quantity. Visually, it looks like this:

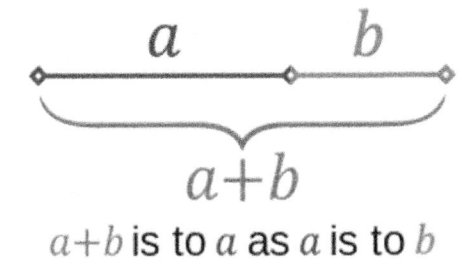

$$\underbrace{\overset{a}{\rule{2cm}{0.4pt}}\overset{b}{\rule{1.2cm}{0.4pt}}}_{a+b}$$

$a+b$ is to a as a is to b

If b measures at 1 unit then a measures at 1.618033999749895...

The Golden Spiral, a manifestation of the Golden Ratio, is an example of sacred geometry in action. From the magnificence of swirling galaxies to the elegance of a nautilus shell, this spiral pattern is a recurring signature of the divine symmetry in nature. It's a visual reminder that the universe operates on principles of harmony and proportion.

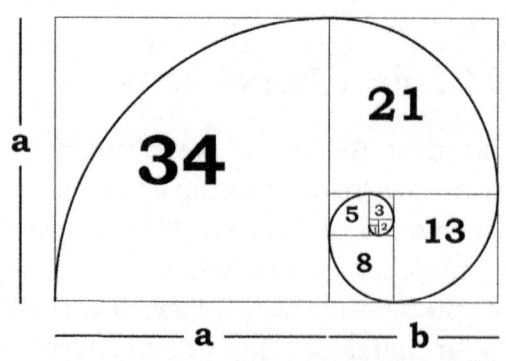

In geometry, a golden spiral is a logarithmic spiral whose growth factor is the golden ratio. That is, a golden spiral gets wider (or further from its origin) by a factor of the golden ratio for every quarter turn it makes.

Artists throughout history have been captivated by this proportion, incorporating it into their masterpieces for thousands of years. They understood, perhaps intuitively, that this ratio represented a form of aesthetic perfection. This concept of ideal proportions was not limited to art; it extended into the realms of architecture and human anatomy.

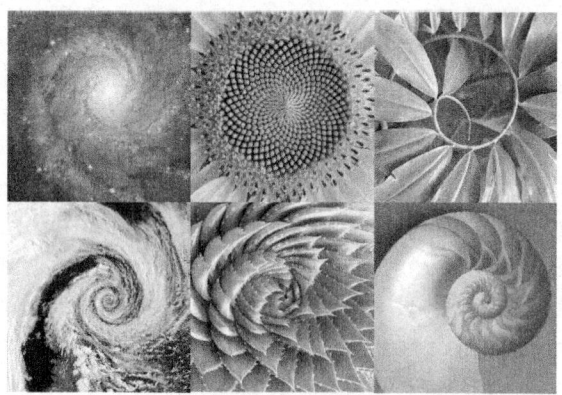

The golden spiral is a universal pattern that occurs across the natural world.

Marcus Vitruvius, a Roman architect during the first century BC, authored an all encompassing guide to classical architectural design titled *De Architectura*. Vitruvius promoted the idea that all buildings should embody *'firmitas'*, *'utilitas'*, and *'venustas'* (strength, utility, and beauty). But he didn't stop at architecture; Vitruvius applied these same principles to the human body. He theorized that the human body itself could model specific proportions that reflect a kind of divine symmetry.

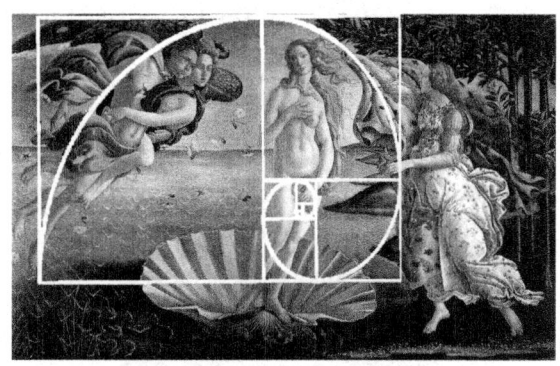

Artists and architects in the Renaissance and ancient Greece were not just creating beauty; they were tapping into sacred geometry.

Inspired by the writings of Vitruvius, Leonardo da Vinci drew the *Vitruvian Man*. Da Vinci's drawing is a tribute to the human form, a blend of art and mathematics, showcasing the body as a mirror of the universal order.

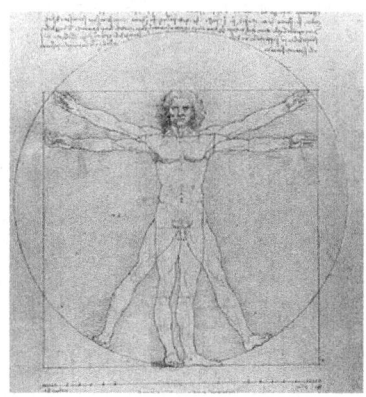

"Man is a model of the world," said Leonardo Da Vinci and his iconic drawing of the Vitruvian Man represents his conception of ideal body proportions.

But the story of the ideal human form doesn't end there. In

ancient Greece, Polykleitos, renowned as a master sculptor of men, studied the mathematics of beauty and wrote a treatise outlining the basis of the ideal male body shape. Although his original writings were lost, his statue *Doryphoros* stands as a testament to his theory of harmonious proportions, embodying the physical manifestation of his mathematical insights.

As we connect these historical dots, from Euclid to Vitruvius, from Leonardo da Vinci to Polykleitos, we see a consistent theme: the pursuit of harmony and proportion, principles that have guided artists, architects, and mathematicians in their quest to capture the essence of beauty.

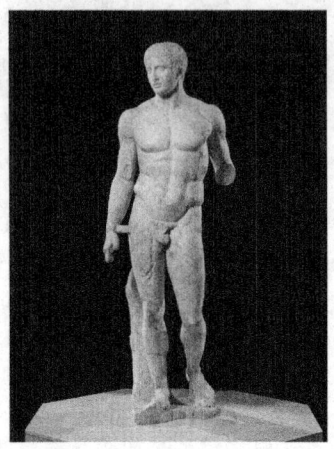

Polykleitos was known in ancient Greece as the best sculptor of men, with the primary subjects of his works being male athletes. He was interested in the mathematical proportions of the human form, which led him to write an essay, the Kanon, on the proportions of humans. The Doryphoros (pictured above) is an illustration of his writings on the symmetry between the body parts.

In the realm of fitness, these ancient principles take on new life. Eugen Sandow, in studying the classical statues and applying these timeless concepts, bridged the gap between the art of the past and the fitness goals of the present. The Golden Ratio, as applied to the human body, is about specific measurements that resonate with a deep, universal aesthetic appeal.

According to the Golden Ratio, the ideal male physique has a shoulder circumference that is 1.618 times the size of the waist. In applying this formula to your own physique, it starts with establishing a reference point for your waist measurement. We want a waist without extra inches of fat. In Chapter 1, we determined the difference between your current and target waist measurement. The standard we're aiming for is a waist that measures at 45% or less of your height. This sets the stage for ideal proportions because carrying excess body fat distorts all your other measurements.

With a lean waist, we turn our attention to the shoulders. The goal here is to achieve a circumference that is 1.618 times greater than your lean waist. This creates the classic V-tapered look, resembling the Greek statues and symbolizing strength and balance.

Getting your shoulder to waist ratio to resemble the Golden Ratio will give your body an attractive, masculine frame. But when it comes to complete development, we need to consider other parts of the body as well.

Balancing The Body: The Reeves Ratios

In the records of bodybuilding history, Eugen Sandow stands as a pioneer, the first man to sculpt his body into a living example of specific proportions. His legacy lives on with his statue atop the 'Sandow Trophy' which is awarded to winners of the Mr. Olympia bodybuilding competitions. Bodybuilding as a sport, however, has evolved drastically over the years, transitioning from a pursuit of aesthetic proportions to a race for sheer muscle size. Amidst this evolution, a different kind of legend emerged in the 1940s — Steve Reeves.

Reeves' name is synonymous with the classic physique. His body appears scrawny when compared to the bodybuilders of today, yet in the 40s he held the titles of Mr. America, Mr. World, and

Mr. Universe before the era of steroids. His physique, unlike the oversized figures of modern bodybuilding, was a harmonious blend of strength and symmetry. It's this enduring appeal of Reeves' form that we can use as a blueprint for timeless aesthetics.

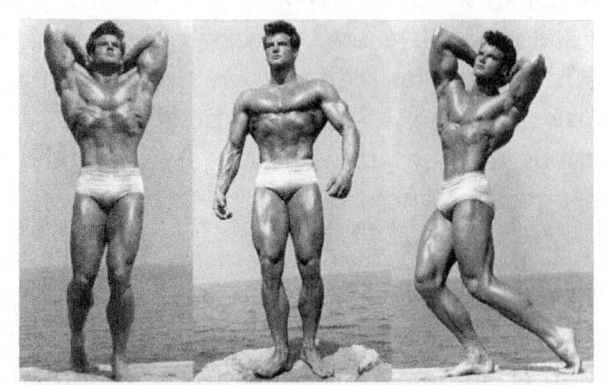

To this day, Steve Reeves maintains a legacy for symmetrical muscle proportions.

In his book *Building the Classic Physique: The Natural Way*, Reeves outlines a series of measurements that form the basis of what I call the 'Reeves Ratios.' These are numbers calculated from reference points of the body, much like how the Golden Ratio uses height and waist as a baseline. For instance, Reeves suggests that the ideal arm size should be 252% of the wrist size, and the ideal calf size matches the arm size, creating a balance that transcends time.

Though Reeves physique is attainable naturally without steroids, each body is unique with its own genetic blueprint. What Reeves provides are guidelines, a north star of balanced aesthetics to steer our fitness journey towards.

Combining Reeves' insights with Sandow's Grecian Ideal and the universal appeal of the Golden Ratio, I've distilled a set of custom ratios that consider the unique dimensions of every individual:

- Arms = 2.5 x wrist

- Calves = arms
- Neck = arms
- Waist = 0.45 x height
- Shoulders = 1.618 x waist
- Thighs = 1.75 x knee
- Chest = 6.5 x wrist

These ratios provide a roadmap to achieving a physique that balances strength with elegance and power with proportion. It's a fusion of historical wisdom and modern understanding, a formula that guides you towards a body with an athletic, aesthetic look.

As we journey further into the art of sculpting your ideal physique, remember, these ratios are tools, not chains. They're meant to inspire, guide, and help you visualize the ideal, while acknowledging and celebrating your body's unique story.

Sculpting Your Masterpiece

In this journey from past to present, we've uncovered the timeless principles that bridge art, history, and bodybuilding. Starting with Eugen Sandow's meticulous study in a museum, we dove into the world of the Golden Ratio and the legacies of Leonardo da Vinci, Polykleitos, and Steve Reeves. These pioneers of proportion have shown us that achieving a physique that is both strong and aesthetically pleasing is an art form in itself.

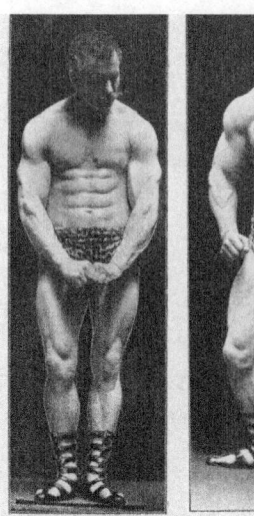

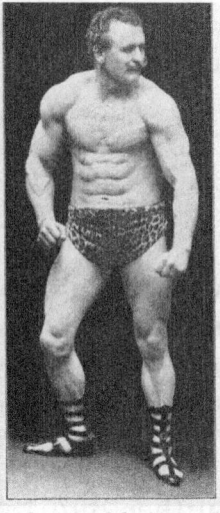

*Long before the invention of steroids, Sandow sculpted
a physique that is revered through the ages.*

Remember, these ratios are flexible tools to guide you on your journey, adaptable to your unique body structure. They offer a path to sculpt body proportions that resonate with a harmony known and admired for centuries.

As we conclude this chapter, let's revisit Sandow in the museum, each measurement he took was a step towards his ideal physique. Your journey, like his, is about transforming theory into a living sculpture. Your body, a canvas for your dedication and hard work.

Equipped with the knowledge of what makes a physique aesthetically pleasing, it's time to proceed towards the fundamental principles that will empower you to achieve these ideals. In the next chapter on *The Five Laws of Lifting*, we will dissect the core tenets of effective strength training.

Prepare to explore the bedrock of functional fitness, where every lift and every rep is a step closer to achieving a harmonious, powerful and capable physique. Turn the page as we deconstruct the laws that will guide your lifting journey, turning your aspirations into tangible reality.

Chapter Takeaways

- Eugen Sandow, the father of bodybuilding, pioneered an approach focused on emulating the 'Grecian Ideal', blending strength with aesthetic proportions derived from classical art.

- The Golden Ratio, discovered by the mathematician Euclid, manifests in the Golden Spiral and sacred geometry, underscoring its importance in art, nature, and human anatomy.

- The works of Vitruvius, Leonardo da Vinci, and Polykleitos in architecture, art, and sculpture demonstrate the enduring application of ideal human proportions and the Golden Ratio.

- Steve Reeves' is a legend in the bodybuilding world from the 40s and 50s who's legacy rests on the balance and symmetry of proportion. His recommended ratios provide a practical framework for achieving a naturally proportionate and aesthetically appealing physique.

- The integration of principles from Sandow, Reeves, and the Golden Ratio offers a modern blueprint for sculpting a balanced and visually pleasing physique.

Success Check-In Exercise

Before moving on, let's take note of your current measurements to determine where you stand. For your limbs take note of both left and right sides to assess imbalances. Next, use the formulas as discussed in this chapter to determine your ideal measurements and compare them to your current form.

Step 1 - Take note of your current waist measurement by

wrapping a tape measure around your torso in the area above your belly button and below your lowest rib. Let your stomach hang in a neutral position rather than sucking it in.

Step 2 - Take note of your current shoulder measurement by having someone wrap a tape measure around your shoulders at the widest point as your arms hang by your side. Write it down in the table below.

Step 3 - Take note of your current chest measurement by having someone wrap a tape measure at the fullest part of your pecs. The tape measure should run under your armpits and across your shoulder blades all the way around your upper body.

Step 4 - Take note of your current arms measurement by wrapping a tape measure around the largest part of your flexed bicep. Do this for both your left and right side body to assess any imbalances.

Step 5 - Take note of your thigh measurement by wrapping a tape measure around the widest part of your flexed leg. Do this for both your left and right side body to assess any imbalances.

Step 6 - Take note of your calf measurement by wrapping a tape measure around the widest part of your flexed calf (i.e. heel raised up off the floor). Do this for both your left and right side body to assess any imbalances.

Step 7 - Take note of your wrist measurement by wrapping a tape measure around the smallest part of your non-dominant wrist while you make a fist with your hand. If you're right handed, measure your left wrist. If you're left handed, measure your right wrist.

Step 8 - Take note of your knee measurement by wrapping a tape measure around the center of your kneecap.

Step 9 - Record all of your measurements in the table below:

	Current	Ideal	Gap
Waist			
Shoulders			
Chest			
Arms	Right: Left:		
Thighs	Right Left		
Calves	Right: Left:		
Wrist		N/A	N/A
Knee		N/A	N/A

Step 10 - Take note of your ideal body measurements by using the formulas outlined in this chapter or referring to the following image.

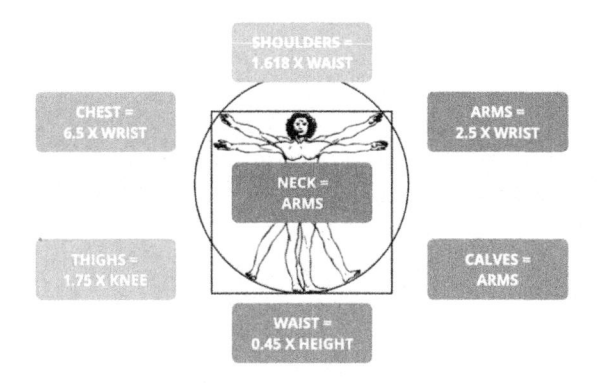

- SHOULDERS = 1.618 X WAIST
- CHEST = 6.5 X WRIST
- ARMS = 2.5 X WRIST
- NECK = ARMS
- THIGHS = 1.75 X KNEE
- CALVES = ARMS
- WAIST = 0.45 X HEIGHT

Step 11 - Determine the gap between your current and ideal measurements and take note in the table above.

It's helpful to think of these ratios as guiding stars rather than awaiting shores. In other words, you may never reach your ideal body but as long as your measurements are moving in the right direction, then that means you're making progress.

CHAPTER 6 - THE FIVE LAWS OF LIFTING

"As to methods, there may be a million and then some, but principles are few. The man who grasps principles can successfully select his own methods. The man who tries methods, ignoring principles, is sure to have trouble."

—HARRINGTON EMMERSON

Picture this: two architects are getting ready to construct their buildings in the middle of a city. One architect starts off fast. He's using all the latest styles and ideas to make his building look modern and fancy. It's exciting, and everyone is talking about it.

Not too far away, there's another architect, but he's doing things differently. Instead of jumping right in, he's spending time looking at old buildings that have lasted for hundreds of years. He wants to know why they're still standing strong. He's digging into history and learning from the past.

The first building goes up quickly. It looks great at first, but then problems start to show. It turns out, the architect focused too much on making it trendy, but not enough on making it strong and lasting.

Meanwhile, the second architect's project is taking more time. He's careful, choosing strong materials and building in a way that's proven to last. His building doesn't just look good; it's built to stand the test of time. This is a lot like fitness where the latest exercise trend or craze gains a lot of attention but the basic, time-tested ways to build a strong, healthy and functional body remain the same.

In this chapter, we're going to deconstruct the principles of long-term strength and vitality. Think of it like learning to architect a building that lasts. I'll show you how to structure your training the right way so you can construct a solid foundation that supports you for a lifetime.

By the end of this chapter, you'll know how to use fundamental principles rather than passing trends to guide your fitness journey.

Let's get started.

The Five Universal Laws Of Training

This chapter is dedicated to uncovering the core principles that are time-tested and universally acknowledged by the most successful practitioners in the realm of physical development. You will learn not about fleeting fitness fads, but about the five universal laws of strength training that remain relevant regardless of whether you're doing calisthenics or any other type of exercise. These principles form a framework that allows you to create a personalized training routine, honed for your unique physique and goals.

By embracing these laws, you can ensure that your efforts are intelligently aligned with the deeper science of human performance. Prepare to elevate your understanding from the conventional to the conceptual, enabling you to navigate the landscape of physical culture with confidence and clarity.

Law #1 - Specificity: Crafting Your Unique Path

If we imagine your fitness journey as a road trip, then the law of specificity is your GPS. Known in the scientific world as SAID, or 'Specific Adaptation to Imposed Demands,' this principle is elegantly straightforward: you reap exactly what you sow in your training.

If you're training to become a sprinter, you wouldn't spend all your time swimming, right? Just as a gardener plants specific seeds for the flowers he wants to grow, your workouts must align precisely with your goals.

The world of fitness, heavily influenced by bodybuilding, often misguides enthusiasts into one-size-fits-all routines. But the truth is that there's no universal routine that works perfectly for everyone.

Throughout this book, I'm making the case for why calisthenics is the supreme style of exercise to achieve the overarching goal of longevity. But maybe your goal is to run a marathon. In that case, your training should focus on long-distance running with an understanding of the downsides. Or maybe your goal is to compete in a powerlifting competition, in which case you should focus on explosive weight lifting with an understanding of the injury risk. See the difference? It's like choosing the right tool for the job - you wouldn't use a hammer to screw in a lightbulb.

The Law of Specificity is the most important principle of training. If your workouts don't align with your goals, it's like trying to navigate a foreign city without a map. You will eventually get somewhere, but it's probably not where you wanted to go.

Law #2 - Progressive Overload: The Art Of Constant Challenge

As you navigate the road trip of your fitness journey, think of progressive overload as the fuel that powers your progress. This fundamental law states that to keep progressing, you need to continuously challenge your body with increased intensity. It's about upping the ante, pushing yourself a bit further each time to keep the progress coming.

Consider the journey of mastering push ups. When you first start, doing a basic push up can be challenging. Your muscles strain, your heart races, and completing a single set is a triumph. But as you practice, your strength and endurance improve, and those same push ups become easier. This is where progressive overload must come into play. To continue advancing, you need to increase the difficulty of the exercise.

But how can we progressively overload with calisthenics when we only have so many pounds of body weight to work with? By decreasing leverage through the redistribution of our body weight between our limbs. For instance, after mastering standard push ups, you can progress to diamond push ups, where your hands form a diamond shape, placing more stress on your triceps. Another step could be elevating your feet, increasing the resistance and working your upper chest and shoulders more intensely. Eventually, you may advance towards single arm push-ups, significantly increasing the load on your muscles with each rep. Each progression represents a step up in difficulty, ensuring that your body is continually being challenged to grow and adapt.

Progressive overload in calisthenics is about creativity and understanding how to modify exercises to increase their intensity. This principle is crucial for continuous improvement. Without it, your progress plateaus and your workouts lose their effectiveness.

As we dive deeper in later chapters, we'll explore various progressions to implement overload in bodyweight exercises. We'll learn how to tweak angles, leverage, and even tempo to keep pushing our limits.

Remember, the essence of progressive overload in calisthenics is advancing through stages, constantly challenging yourself with more complex or demanding variations of exercises. It's this continual push that fuels your journey towards greater strength and an ever-improving physique.

Law #3 - Individuality: Your Custom Fitness Vehicle

As you journey along the fitness highway, the Law of Individuality serves as the blueprint for customizing your vehicle – your training program. This law states that your approach to fitness should suit your individual situation. It's about understanding that the path for a seasoned athlete is vastly different from the path a beginner takes.

This law stands in contrast to the 'one-size-fits-all' plans found online. Your fitness program should be as unique as your fingerprint, crafted to fit your personal abilities and experience level. For instance, a program that suits you now, with specific objectives and at your current experience level, will evolve over time as you progress.

Furthermore, two individuals with the same destination in mind will still require different routes. A beginner just starting out needs a different approach compared to a seasoned veteran who has been on the road for years. The difference in their training isn't determined by the destination they aim for but by the paths they need to take based on their individual starting points.

In essence, the Law of Individuality states that your fitness program must be tailored to you as an individual. Whether your goals align with those of others or differ entirely, your training plan must adjust to your unique abilities, needs, and aspirations.

As we continue to explore the Laws of Lifting, remember that your fitness journey is yours alone. It's a road trip where the route, the scenery, and the pace are all yours to determine. Embrace the uniqueness of your journey, and let the Law of Individuality guide you in creating a training program that's perfectly suited for you, ensuring a journey that's not only effective but also enjoyable and fulfilling.

Law #4 - Maintenance: Sustaining Your Gains

In the grand adventure of your fitness journey, reaching your peak fitness goals is like arriving at a breathtaking summit. The Law of Maintenance is what allows you to enjoy the view from the top with less effort than it took to climb. Maintenance is about finding the right balance to sustain your achievements without the intensity of the initial ascent.

Imagine your training as a vehicle that's powered you up a steep hill. Reaching the peak is a tremendous achievement, but the effort needed to stay at the summit is less than the energy it took to get there. Once you're satisfied with your strength levels, it's like reaching a plateau where the road evens out. Here, you can ease off the accelerator, reducing the intensity and frequency of your training sessions. This doesn't mean you stop moving. Instead, you shift gears to maintain your gains while exploring new paths. It's the perfect time to turn your focus to other fitness dimensions like mobility and stamina. Think of it as taking a scenic route; you're still on your fitness journey, but you're now enjoying different aspects of the landscape.

For example, if you've achieved the muscle size or strength you desire, you might reduce the number of strength training sessions and incorporate more mobility or endurance training into your routine, adding variety while keeping your body engaged and active.

The Law of Maintenance underscores an important aspect of fitness: reaching your goal isn't the end of the road. It's a transition to a new phase of your journey, where the emphasis shifts from building to sustaining. This phase allows you to enjoy the results of your hard work and gives you the freedom to explore other fitness areas, adding to your overall well-being.

As we continue exploring the Laws of Lifting, remember that the Law of Maintenance is your companion for the long haul. It ensures that your journey is sustainable and enjoyable, allowing you to cruise comfortably at your fitness peak while keeping your body healthy and active.

Law #5 - Reversibility: Use It Or Lose It

As we reach the final stretch of our exploration, the Law of Reversibility stands as a crucial reminder. On your fitness road trip, if you stop driving altogether, you'll start rolling back down the hill you've worked so hard to climb.

This law highlights a simple yet vital truth: the progress you've made through training is not permanent if left unattended. It's like having your vehicle in neutral on a slope; without some forward momentum, gravity takes over, and you begin to lose ground. In the context of fitness, if you stop training, or if your training falls below an effective threshold, the progress you've made will begin to reverse.

Consider your hard-earned strength or stamina as a campfire that you've built on your journey. If you stop adding wood to the fire, it doesn't stay the same; it slowly dies out. Similarly, your fitness gains require a consistent 'fuel' of exercise to maintain their intensity and benefits.

However, the silver lining of the Law of Reversibility is the Law of Maintenance—it doesn't demand the same level of effort to maintain your gains as it did to achieve them initially. You can think of it as needing to maintain a steady, gentle pressure on the accelerator to keep your vehicle moving forward, rather than the full-throttle effort needed during your initial climb.

To prevent the rollback of your results, it's essential to keep up with a minimum effective dose of exercise. This could be a scaled-back version of your more intensive workout routine or a consistent, moderate level of activity that keeps the engine of your fitness running.

As we wrap up our journey through the Laws of Lifting, remember that the Law of Reversibility doesn't mean you can never take a break. Instead, it's a call to find a sustainable pace that allows you to maintain your fitness achievements and enjoy the long, rewarding drive on the road of health and fitness towards longevity.

Mastery Over Method

True mastery in your fitness journey will come from understanding principles, not merely adopting methods. With the five Laws of Lifting firmly in your toolkit, you're no longer wandering aimlessly in the ever-changing landscape of fitness trends. Instead, you're equipped with a compass of principles, guiding you through the terrain of physical well-being with clarity and purpose.

The power of specificity, the necessity of progressive overload, the wisdom of individuality, the strategy of maintenance, and the caution of reversibility. These laws give you the power to become the architect of your own fitness so you can construct a routine that resonates with your life's rhythm and ambitions.

Your approach to fitness will no longer be swayed by the

latest fads; instead, it will be anchored in timeless principles that hold true regardless of the latest trends. Similar to how a scientist derives laws from careful experiments — your fitness strategy is now grounded in enduring truths that are universally applicable.

As we set our sights on the next chapter, we'll unlock the hidden key to long-term success with calisthenics. You'll also discover the specific mobility exercises that create alignment in your body so you can move freely without pain. You can pick and choose from these exercises according to your specific weak links and where you need to focus.

With these foundational principles firmly established, the path ahead is full of potential and discovery. It's time to dive deeper into the world of calisthenics, armed with the power of principle-driven practice.

Remember, understanding the principles is key; like a compass in the wilderness, they will keep you from running in circles and guide you towards true progress and mastery in your fitness quest.

Chapter Takeaways

- The Law of Specificity ensures that you're navigating through a program that is specifically designed for your goals.

- The Law of Progressive Overload necessitates the continual increase of exercise intensity to keep progressing.

- The Law of Individuality ensures that your program is tailored to your personal abilities and situation.

- The Law of Maintenance allows for sustaining fitness peaks with less effort than the initial climb.

- The Law of Reversibility warns that progress will start to fade if training is stopped, similar to rolling back down a hill, and emphasizing the importance of a minimum effective dose of exercise to retain progress.

- Mastery in fitness comes from understanding and applying principles, not just adopting methods, so you can be an architect of your own fitness journey, charting a course based on enduring principles rather than transient trends.

CHAPTER 7 - CREATING ALIGNMENT PART I

"When your body is not aligned, the inner power will not come. When you are not tranquil within, your mind will not be well ordered. Align your body, assist the inner power, then it will gradually come on its own."

—ZHENG MANQING

P op

The unmistakable sound of my own body failing me— a sound that would echo in my mind long after the initial shock had faded. I was mid-squat, a loaded barbell pressing down on my back, when my knee buckled beneath me. In that split second, before the sharp pain shot through my leg, there was a moment of disbelief. Could this really be happening?

An MRI scan confirmed my fears: a torn lateral meniscus. The cartilage meant to stabilize my knee had been compromised. Surgery was the immediate recommendation from doctors, along with the promise of six to eight months for recovery.

I found myself at a crossroads and began to wonder: Could I trust my body to heal on its own, or would I be living with pain indefinitely if I refused the operation? With these questions swirling in my mind, I started researching arthroscopic surgery, which was the procedure my doctor had recommended. That's when I came across a study that would shift everything for me.

Published in the New England Journal of Medicine in 2013, the study revealed that patients who underwent real arthroscopic surgery for knee pain experienced outcomes almost identical to those who underwent a sham surgery, where their knee was opened up and closed back up again without the actual procedure[8]. In both cases, patients reported similar levels of pain relief and functional improvement. This was a revelation. If surgery didn't offer any real advantage over the body's natural ability to heal, then why take on the risks? In that moment, I made the decision to pursue a path of healing without invasive intervention. It wasn't going to be easy, but I knew it was the right path for me.

After six weeks of physiotherapy, I was back in the gym. My knee hadn't fully healed—I couldn't run, play sports, or hike—but I got back to lifting weights, ignoring the lingering instability. In my mind, I was doing what I needed to get back to strength, but in reality, I was setting myself up for another fall. Lessons we don't learn in life are often repeated and, as fate would have it, my other knee went through a similar story two years later with a tear of its own—a mirror image of neglect. This time, it was more than an injury; it was a wake-up call.

As I lay there, grappling with the frustration and vulnerability of another injury, I arrived at a painful realization:

The body I was training so diligently for strength had, paradoxically, become a display of weakness.

Determined to find a better way, I embarked on yet another journey of research, recovery, and revelation. I dove deep into the study of exercise science and human anatomy, looking to understand the root cause of my injuries. I consulted with chiropractors, physiotherapists, and sports injury specialists, each offering insights that chipped away at my old beliefs. However, it wasn't until I discovered the work of Ben Patrick, founder of Athletic Truth Group, that I experienced a lasting breakthrough.

◆ ◆ ◆

After my second injury, I became overly cautious and steered clear of anything that could possibly aggravate my knees. I stopped playing sports like soccer which was especially difficult because it was the main social activity in my friends' group. I attempted to join a game once, only to quit within ten minutes because even a slight run triggered pain. A single jump while shooting a basketball left me in discomfort for weeks. The fact that I couldn't engage in the very activities I loved was not only frustrating but also depressing. I felt fragile, as though my body had betrayed me.

Desperate for a solution, I came across a video of Ben Patrick (aka knees over toes guy). He was doing what seemed like dangerous exercises that went against everything I believed at the time. I heard him say that, "The athlete whose knees can go farthest and strongest over his toes is the most protected against injury." Up until this point, I had taken an avoidant approach, staying away from exercises that put any strain on my knees, especially those that caused my knees to move beyond my toes.

Ben's approach challenged everything I thought I knew about pain and recovery. He didn't view pain as an enemy to be avoided but as a signal—an indication that something needed attention. He said that icing, painkillers, and other quick fixes were like telling your body to "shut up" when it was trying to communicate a problem. Instead of merely alleviating the symptom, which was pain, Ben's system focused on increasing ability. By starting below my pain threshold and gradually progressing range of motion, I learned that pain could be reduced as a natural byproduct of increasing ability. He explained that while there is pressure on the knee joint when the knees go over the toes, this pressure is safely managed if the muscles and connective tissues around the knee are properly mobilized. The more mobility you build, the more resilient your joints become.

Through this journey, I arrived at a truth that I am compelled to share with you now:

Musculoskeletal alignment is the key that unlocks pain-free movement and protection against injury.

The musculoskeletal system is the body's framework that helps us move and stay upright. It includes bones, muscles, joints, tendons, and ligaments. Bones give our body structure and protect our organs, while muscles work with bones to help us move. Joints are where two bones meet and allow for movement, tendons connect muscles to bones, and ligaments connect bones to each other, keeping everything in place. Together, they make sure we can move, lift, and perform physical activity.

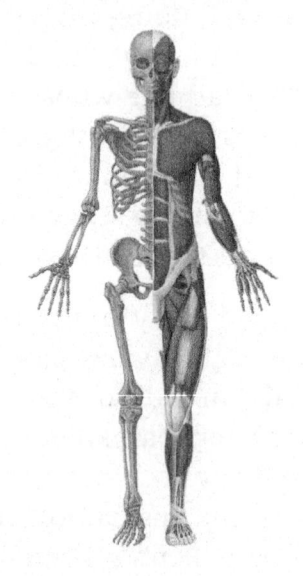

The musculoskeletal system is like the body's framework and engine. Your bones are the structure, your muscles are the motors, your joints are the hinges, and your tendons and ligaments are the connectors and stabilizers. All these parts work together to let you move, lift, run, jump, and perform your daily activities.

Musculoskeletal alignment refers to the optimal positioning and functioning of the bones, muscles, tendons, ligaments, and joints. When these elements are aligned, they work in harmony, distributing stress and strain as nature intended. But when alignment is lost, certain parts of the body compensate to maintain balance and allow for movement. While this compensation can keep you functioning in the short term, it often leads to overuse or strain in those compensating areas. This uneven stress can wear down cartilage, strain ligaments, or cause muscle imbalances, making certain areas more prone to pain and injury.

Looking back, I realize that my bodybuilding-inspired approach to fitness had been a recipe for disaster. I focused on building muscle through isolation exercises, which led to strong muscles but underdeveloped joints and connective tissues. My hips and ankles, in particular, lacked the mobility needed to stabilize my knees. Weak stabilizers coupled with a restricted range of motion forced my knees to compensate, pushing them into vulnerable positions and, ultimately, leading to torn cartilage—a painful lesson in the importance of balance and alignment.

As a coach, I've seen this story play out in many of my clients. Shoulder impingement, lower back pain, shin splints—all too often, the root cause can be traced back to a lack of alignment. When we address these issues through proper mobility training, the pain disappears, and the body regains its natural, pain-free movement.

The implications are clear:

When your mobility is good, your body works efficiently,

minimizing the risk of pain and injury. When mobility is poor, your body can fall out of alignment, leading to compensations that can cause problems down the line.

This chapter is more than a reflection on past mistakes; it's a guide built from them. You will gain the crucial understanding of how to properly mobilize, balance, and align your musculoskeletal system so you can move freely without pain and remain resilient against injury.

As someone who has experienced firsthand the consequences of neglecting alignment, I am deeply passionate about sharing this knowledge with you. This isn't just about avoiding injuries; it's about building a foundation that supports your body's natural mechanics so you can approach your fitness goals with confidence.

Building From The Ground Up

Imagine watching the construction of a skyscraper. Before the steel beams rise, before the glass windows reflect the sky, the builders dig deep into the earth. The taller the building, the deeper they must dig. This foundation is the bedrock that determines the strength, stability, and longevity of the entire structure. Your body is no different.

Starting from your feet and working upwards through your ankles, knees and hips—building from the ground up means aligning with the force of gravity. Gravity constantly pulls your body downward toward the earth and the parts of your body closer to the ground bear more of the force, especially when you're standing, walking, running, or jumping. Because these lower parts of the body are subjected to greater forces, they must be strong enough to handle the stress without causing pain or injury.

The mistake that many people, including myself, have made is building from the top down, prioritizing the aesthetics of the upper body over the foundational mobility of the lower body. In my early days of training, I was drawn to the allure of a broad chest and bulging biceps—muscles that were visible, impressive, and, in my mind, the markers of strength. But like a skyscraper built on shallow ground, this approach left me vulnerable. My upper body may have looked strong, but it rested on a foundation that was shaky and unbalanced. This imbalance contributed to my knee injuries because my body was out of alignment with an overdeveloped torso and underdeveloped legs, leaving me "gravity bound."

Your body's joints are like links in a chain, each one affecting the others. The force acting upon these links is strongest in the lower body, where gravity exerts the most pressure. Therefore, it's crucial to focus on building from the ground up, ensuring that your lower body is well-prepared to handle the forces it encounters.

Throughout the rest of this chapter, I'll guide you through specific exercises to mobilize your feet, ankles, and knees. From there, we'll proceed towards the hips and spine. And in the next chapter, we'll discuss specific mobility exercises for the upper body. By building your body from the ground up, you'll create a balanced foundation that aligns your entire structure and helps prevent injuries.

I learned about the concept of 'building the body from the ground up' from Ben Patrick. For those who are interested in learning more about Ben's work, I recommend securing a copy of his book: *Knee Ability Zero*.

Mobility Exercises For The Feet, Ankles, & Knees

Our feet, ankles, and knees form the foundational pillars of movement, working in harmony to support and propel the body through space. These three areas are crucial not only for balance and stability but also for maintaining alignment throughout the rest of the body. When these areas are mobile, they create a base that protects the joints and tissues above them, ensuring that our movements remain pain-free.

Backward Walking

If you've ever visited a park in China or other parts of Asia, you might have noticed groups of elderly people walking backward. This practice might seem unusual at first, but it's deeply rooted in traditional health practices that have been passed down for generations. Backward walking, or "retro-walking," has been a staple in Asian cultures for thousands of years, recognized for its unique ability to promote joint health and prevent ailments like arthritis. Chinese wisdom even suggests that "a hundred steps backward are worth a thousand steps forward," a saying that highlights the powerful benefits of this simple yet effective movement.

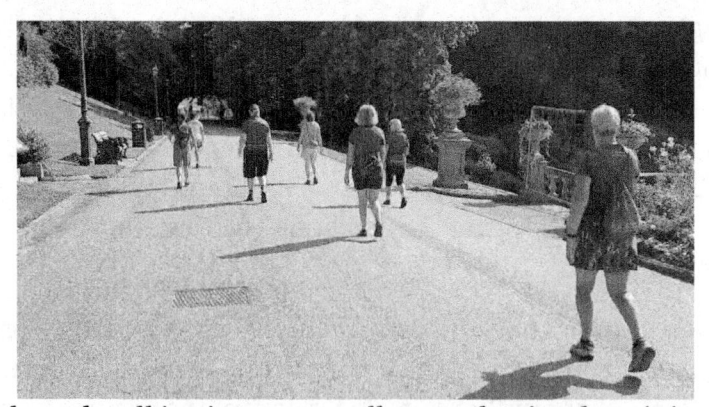

Backward walking is common all around Asia where it is seen as a healing and protective practice for joint health.

Backward walking is an exceptional exercise for improving foot and ankle function. Each step backward requires you to push through your toes, activating the entire foot structure in a way that traditional forward walking does not. This unique movement helps balance foot strength with thigh strength, addressing common issues like plantar fasciitis, shin splints, and Achilles tendinitis. By landing with your foot behind your knee and pushing through with each step, you effectively load the lower leg muscles, building resilience and correcting imbalances that often lead to chronic pain.

On an anatomical level, backward walking stimulates muscles and tendons in areas that are crucial for knee protection, especially compared to forward walking. The vastus medialis muscles—the teardrop-shaped part of your quadriceps near your knees—are particularly engaged when you walk backward. These muscles are the most fast-twitch of your quadriceps, meaning they react quickly to protect your knees and help maintain that spring in your step, which can diminish with age. According to Ben Patrick, "When people with knee pain walk forward, the vastus medialis does not engage like it does for someone without knee pain. But when people with knee pain walk backward, the vastus medialis does engage as it's intended to! So you really can work your way backward to a more protected knee going forward."

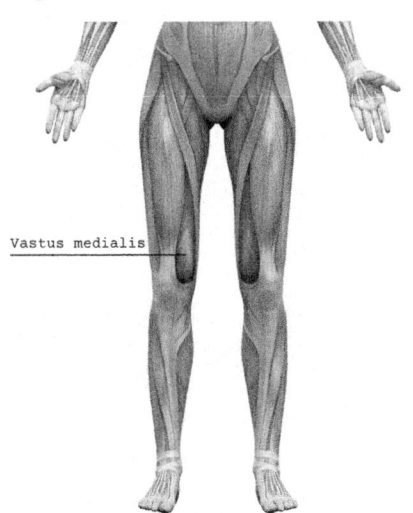

Your vastus medialis muscles are the lower, teardrop-shaped quadricep (thigh) muscles that protect your knees and add that bounce factor we lose as we age.

My journey with backward walking began after my series of

knee injuries left me searching for a way to stay active without pain. After my second injury, I turned to yoga and Qigong, which offered some relief. Feeling encouraged, I ventured into kickboxing, only to have the knee pain resurface. Thankfully, I avoided further injury, but the discomfort was a clear sign that I needed to find a better solution.

Religiously incorporating backward walking into my routine is what allowed me to rebuild resilience in my knees and address foot issues that had been lingering for years. As a result, I was able to start training combat sports consistently without knee pain and even competed in my first Mixed martial arts (MMA) competition—something I had been dreaming about for years.

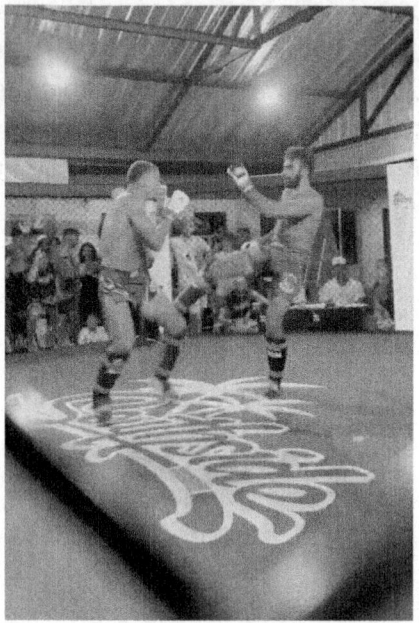

Backward walking, an ancient practice with modern benefits, continues to support my ongoing athletic journey. Without it, I would not have been able to start training combat sports.

Incorporating backward walking into your routine can be done:

- On a treadmill that's turned off so you push through your feet to spin it in reverse

- Using a sled with additional weight to add resistance and intensity, or
- By going up a steep hill

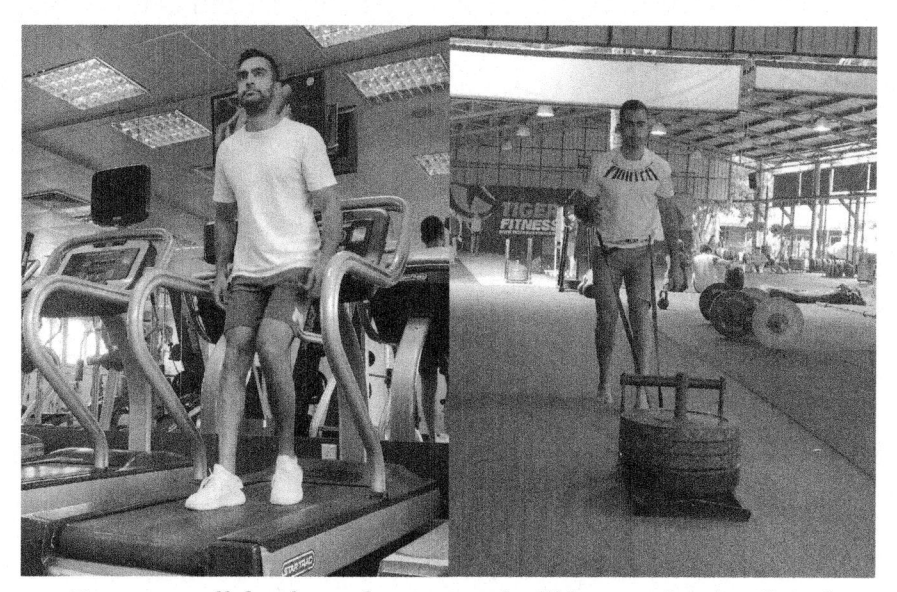

You can walk backward on a treadmill by turning it off and spinning it in reverse or with additional resistance attached to a sled. But equipment is not necessary to get started.

To this day, I incorporate backward walking as a warm up before my workouts. I set a timer for 5 minutes and walk backward at a regular pace for 4 minutes. For the last minute, I jog/run backward as fast as I can. In the beginning, I walked backward without added resistance on a flat surface. As I got stronger, I added resistance on a sled. When traveling, I seek out steep hills that I can run up in reverse, ensuring that there is no incoming traffic and that I have a solid grip. If I'm lucky enough to stay at hotels with a gym, I hop onto a treadmill and spin it in reverse. So there are many options to choose from depending on your level and what you have access to.

Tibialis Raise

This simple exercise directly targets the tibialis anterior muscle which plays a crucial role in foot stability, ankle mobility, and lower leg resilience. This muscle is often overlooked in traditional training programs, leading to imbalances and, ultimately, injury.

With every step, jump, or sudden stop, the tibialis anterior is responsible for flexing your toes upward and decelerating your foot as it makes contact with the ground. As such, the tibialis anterior serves as your body's first line of defense against lower body injuries.

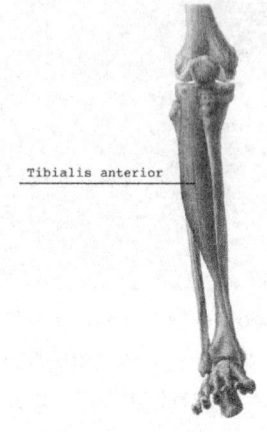

Your tibialis anterior is the muscle that runs along the front of your shin, starting just below your knee and wrapping down to attach inside your foot.

A lot of injuries in sports happen during deceleration—the very moment\ when your body has to absorb and control the force of movement. Think about the force that goes through your body when you land from a jump or make a sudden stop. In high-impact sports, this force can amount to thousands of pounds. When the tibialis is strong, it absorbs and distributes the force that would otherwise transfer to your knees and other joints, reducing the risk of injury. If this muscle is underdeveloped, however, the stress it fails to manage goes directly to your knees, increasing the likelihood of pain and injury.

Steps to Perform the Tibialis Raise:

- Setup:
    1. Stand with your glutes placed against a wall (or sturdy surface) and your heels about 6-12 inches away from the wall. The further your heels are from the wall, the more intense this exercise becomes.
    2. Your heels should be planted firmly on the ground with your legs straight.
    3. Keep your body upright and your back leaning slightly forward.
    4. Feet should be a couple inches apart, and your toes should point forward.

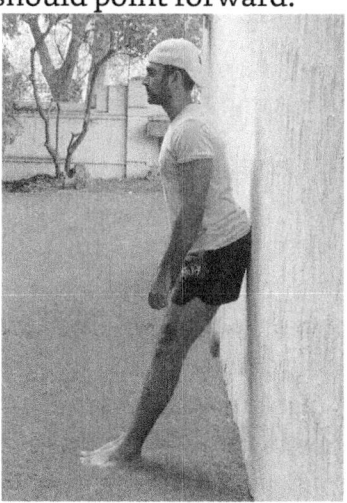

- Execution:
    1. Lift your toes up toward your shins, keeping your heels in contact with the ground. Hold the top position for 1-2 seconds. The movement should be slow and controlled, engaging your tibialis anterior.

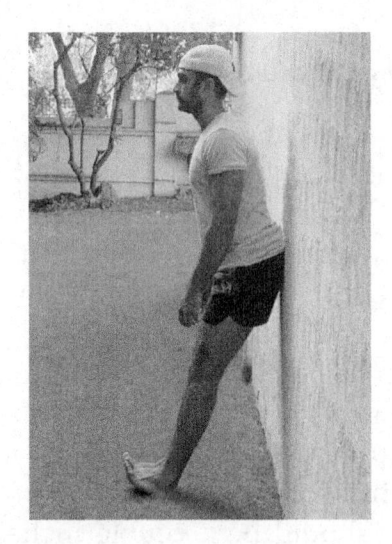

- Follow-through:
    1. Slowly lower your toes back down, avoiding any quick or jerky movements.
    2. Repeat for reps.

By consistently practicing the tibialis raise, you will not only improve ankle mobility and foot control but also reduce the risk of shin splints, a common issue for athletes. Strengthening your tibialis anterior will give you better control over your foot placement and enhance your ability to decelerate safely. This is particularly important as we age and the body's natural elasticity starts to diminish. By fortifying the muscles and tendons that bear the brunt of our movements, we can move freely, with less pain, and continue to pursue our athletic goals without the constant fear of injury.

Fhl Calf Raise

When it comes to lower body development, the focus often remains on larger muscles like the quads and calves. However, there's a smaller, yet equally vital muscle that plays a crucial role in stabilizing the foot and ankle—the flexor hallucis longus (FHL). Running from your big toe up to your mid-calf, the FHL is integral to maintaining balance and control, especially when weight is distributed onto the ball of your foot. This muscle not only supports big toe flexion but also provides stability to the ankle, making it an essential component in your body's overall defense system during movement.

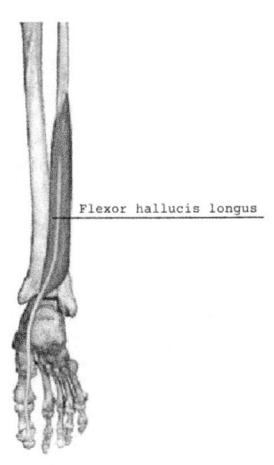

Your FHL muscle starts in the back part of your lower leg and runs down the inside through the ankle, attaching to the bottom of your big toe.

The FHL calf raise is an exercise that directly targets this often-overlooked muscle, offering benefits that extend beyond traditional calf raises. While regular calf raises certainly have their place in a well-rounded fitness routine, they tend to neglect the big toe's involvement, which is crucial for proper foot mechanics. The FHL calf raise emphasizes the role of the big toe, enhancing its flexion and, as a byproduct, improving overall foot and ankle mobility.

Steps to Perform FHL Calf Raise:

- Setup:
    1. Stand facing a wall (or sturdy surface) and place your hands against it at shoulder height.
    2. Step back from the wall until your feet are stretched far enough that your heels rise slightly

off the ground. You should feel a stretch in your calves. Your body should be in a straight line from head to heels, with your arms supporting you against the wall. Your legs should be straight, without bending your knees or hips.

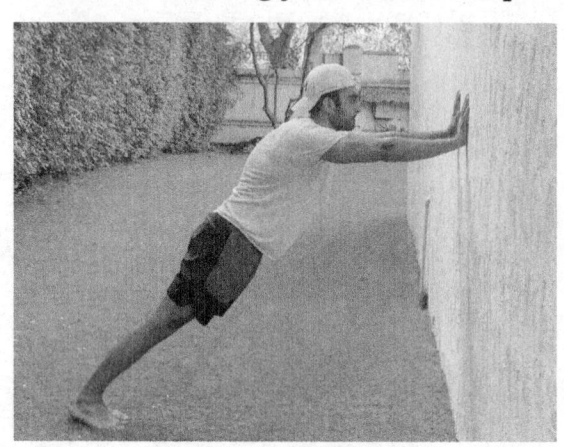

- Execution:
    1. Lift your heels up, transferring your weight onto the balls of your feet with a focus on pushing through your big toes.
    2. As you rise, keep your knees straight and avoid breaking at the hips. The movement should come entirely from the ankle joint, ensuring the FHL muscle (which helps flex the big toe) is fully engaged. You should feel the contraction in your calves and the muscles of your feet, particularly around the big toe area.
    3. Hold the top position for 1-2 seconds.

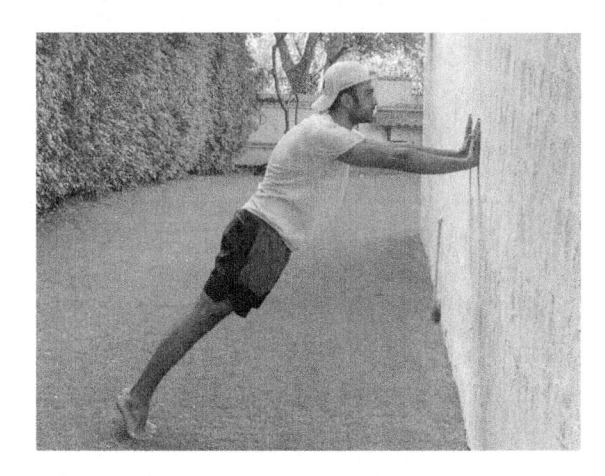

- Follow-through:
    1. Slowly lower your heels back down to the starting position, but don't let them fully rest on the ground—maintain that slight off-the-ground position to keep tension on the calves and FHL.
    2. Repeat for reps.

Incorporating the FHL calf raise into your routine does more than just strengthen the foot; it also promotes a deeper stretch in the ankle, which is vital for maintaining mobility and preventing common issues like Achilles tendonitis and plantar fasciitis. This exercise provides a unique combination of strengthening and stretching, targeting the lower leg muscles that are directly involved in deceleration and landing mechanics. Just as the tibialis raise serves as your first line of defense against lower body injuries during deceleration, the FHL calf raise acts as a protective mechanism when landing.

Every time you land from a jump or step onto uneven terrain, your FHL muscle works to stabilize your ankle and foot, absorbing impact and preventing excessive strain from reaching your knees and hips. The importance of this muscle cannot be overstated—when it's weak or underdeveloped, the force that isn't managed by the FHL travels upward, potentially leading to knee pain and injuries. By building strength in this critical area, you're laying the groundwork for better foot mechanics, which supports your entire kinetic chain.

As I learned from my experience with knee injuries, neglecting the smaller muscles in your lower legs can have significant consequences. Since incorporating the FHL calf raise into my training, I've noticed a marked improvement in both my ankle mobility and overall lower leg strength. This exercise, like the others we've discussed, is essential for anyone looking to build an injury-resistant lower body.

Patrick Step

When it comes to preventing knee injuries, the key often lies in the ability of your knees to move beyond your toes with control. The farther and stronger your knees can travel in this direction, the more protected they are against injury. However, for many of us, especially those recovering from knee issues, this range of motion is not something we start with. I personally experienced significant pain whenever I tried to move my knees even slightly beyond my toes after my injury. Enter the Patrick step—this gentle exercise, named after the man himself, Ben Patrick, is designed to help you progressively develop this crucial ability.

The Patrick step involves stepping forward with control, allowing your knee to glide over your toes while maintaining balance and stability. It's a foundational exercise in building the stability and mobility needed to protect and even heal your knees from injury.

As you gradually improve in this exercise, you'll notice a reduction in knee pain and a significant increase in your overall knee resilience. The Patrick step doesn't just stop at the knees; it also targets your ankle mobility. The more control and strength your ankle has in a bent position, the more effectively it can absorb force and prevent it from transferring up to the knee.

This exercise is especially important for anyone looking to

return to high-impact sports or activities after an injury. By training your knees and ankles to handle the forces that come with deep bends and forward movement, you're laying the groundwork for long-term joint health and stability. In my own journey back to pain-free movement, incorporating the Patrick step was a game-changer—it allowed me to regain confidence in my knee's ability to move safely over my toes without pain.

Steps to Perform Patrick Step:

- Setup:
    1. Place one foot flat on an elevated platform or step that is 2-6 inches high. The higher the platform, the higher the intensity. Your other foot should be off the platform, hovering above the ground. This foot will remain off the ground during the exercise.

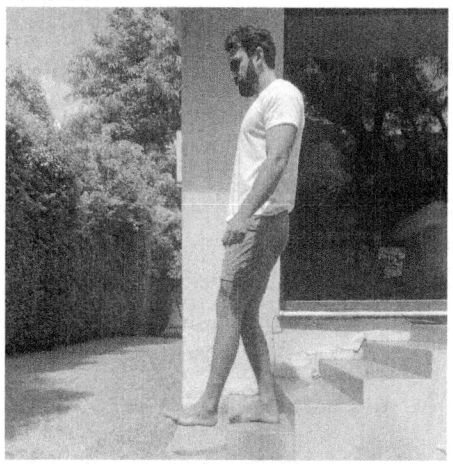

- Execution:
    1. Initiate the downward motion by bending the knee of the foot on the platform.
    2. As you lower, your heel on the working leg should stay flat on the platform, and your knee should track over your toes.
    3. The non-working leg (the one off the platform) should descend toward the ground. Aim to lightly

tap the heel of this foot on the ground without shifting your weight onto it.

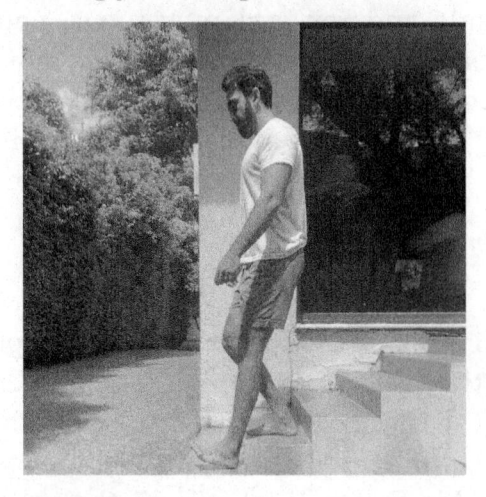

- Follow-through:
    1. Once you've reached the bottom of your range, press through the foot on the platform to return to the starting position.
    2. Repeat for reps.

The Patrick step is a progressive exercise, meaning you start with a manageable range of motion and gradually increase the distance your knee travels over your toes as your ankle mobility and knee stability improve. This controlled progression ensures that you're not overloading your joints too quickly, which is essential for avoiding setbacks during recovery.

For those dealing with knee pain or recovering from an injury, the Patrick step offers a safe and effective way to rebuild the mobility needed for pain-free movement. As you master this exercise, you'll find that not only do your knees become more resilient, but your overall lower body stability improves as well, reducing the risk of injury across the board.

By focusing on the health and mobility of your feet, ankles, and knees, you create a solid foundation that supports the rest of your body. Addressing these areas not only reduces the risk of injury but also enhances your ability to perform complex movements with confidence and ease. Whether you're an athlete looking to optimize performance or someone seeking to improve everyday movement, these exercises are essential steps in your journey to long-term fitness success.

Programming For The Feet, Ankles & Knees

There are many different ways to program the above four exercises. You can perform them in a circuit style workout on its own, you can use them as a warmup before your main workout, you can perform them as a finisher to your main workout, you can pick and choose individual exercises to include in your main workout, and so on. When I was recovering from my knee injuries, I performed the exercises one after the other in a circuit workout 2-3 times per week.

SAMPLE FOOT, ANKLE, AND KNEE WORKOUT

1. **Backward walking: 5-10 minutes**

Perform at a regular pace and then finish with 2-3 minutes going as fast as possible.

2. **Tibialis raise: 2-3 sets x 15-25 reps**

Perform exercises 2-4 in a circuit, i.e. one after the other with minimal break between exercises and 1-3 minute rest between rounds.

3. **FHL calf raise: 2-3 sets x 15-25 reps**

4. **Patrick step: 2-3 sets x 15-25 reps**

This approach isn't set in stone. Experiment to see what works best for you and then select an approach that supports your situation and goals.

Mobility Exercises For The Hips & Spine

Our hips and spine form the central axis of our body, acting as the bridge between the lower and upper halves of the musculoskeletal system. The hips are what allow us to transfer force efficiently from the legs into the rest of the body, while the spine maintains our posture, supports the weight of the upper body, and enables dynamic movement.

Proper alignment and mobility in the hips and spine are essential for maintaining balance and fluidity throughout the kinetic chain. When these areas are mobile, they not only safeguard the joints and tissues of the lower back, but they also ensure that the entire body can move freely without risk of injury.

By targeting the hips and spine, the following exercises will help improve range of motion, reduce stiffness, and create a strong foundation for transferring force throughout the body. Mobilizing these key regions will not only support proper posture and spinal health but also ensure that your entire body moves efficiently and pain-free, optimizing both performance and injury prevention.

Deep Squat Hold

The deep squat hold, where your hamstrings rest on your calves and your hips sink below your knees, is more than just an exercise—it's an expression of primal human mobility and a vital movement pattern deeply ingrained in our evolutionary history. This position is a natural litmus test for the functional range of motion in your hips, knees, ankles, and pelvic muscles, requiring balance, stability, and integrated strength throughout the lower body. It's also a direct reflection of how aligned and mobile your body remains.

In many parts of the world, particularly in less industrialized societies, the deep squat remains a standard resting posture, used for everything from eating to working. In fact, this archetypal position is hardwired into our DNA, revealing its deep physiological significance. The developing joints of a human fetus are primed for this deep squat range of motion, and if you observe a toddler, you'll see them effortlessly dropping into a perfect squat to pick things up off the floor. This illustrates that our bodies are designed to squat deeply, without restriction, from birth.

Zoologist Jonathan Kingdon, in his book *Lowly Origins*, describes the deep squat as an evolutionary pre-adaptation that allowed early humans to maintain a straight spine while working or eating from the ground. Before humans evolved to walk upright, squatting was a foundational movement that shaped our joints and musculature. In this way, the deep squat acts as a reset for the body—a way to restore natural movement patterns that are often neglected in modern life.

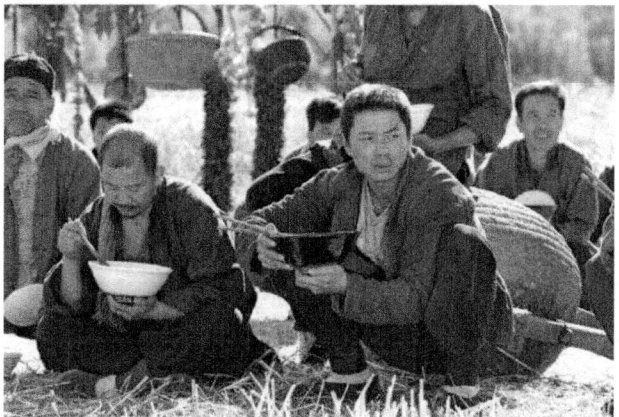

The deep squat is often called an Asian squat because it is a common resting position across many Asian cultures.

In modern society, however, the deep squat is a position that many have lost the ability to enter. Prolonged sitting in chairs has replaced this natural movement pattern, limiting our mobility and gradually disrupting the body's harmony. Years of restricted motion from sitting not only tighten the muscles around the hips, knees, and ankles but also contribute to poor posture and stiffness in the spine.

Regular practice of the deep squat offers a powerful method for regaining mobility in the hips, knees, and ankles, while also improving spinal alignment. By sinking into this position, you engage and stretch multiple muscle groups, including the quads, hamstrings, glutes, and hip flexors. Simultaneously, the position challenges the mobility of the ankles and promotes lengthening and decompression of the spine. Over time, this practice can restore natural functionality to your joints, detoxify metabolic byproducts, and improve overall stability and flexibility.

Steps to Perform a Deep Squat Hold:

- Setup:
    1. Start by taking a light hop off the floor with both feet and notice where they land—this will likely be your natural stance for the deep squat.
    2. Your feet should be about shoulder-width apart with toes pointing slightly outward.

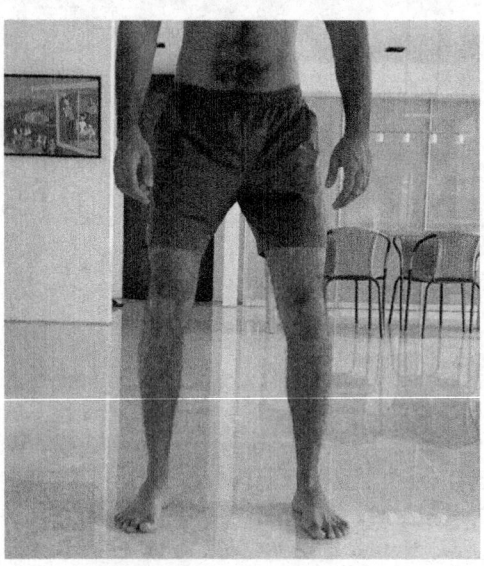

- Execution:
    1. As you lower, focus on keeping your chest up and your spine in a neutral position, avoiding any excessive rounding of the back.
    2. Continue descending until your hamstrings rest on your calves and your hips are fully below your knees. In this bottom position, your knees should track over your toes and avoid letting them cave inward.
    3. Keep your weight evenly distributed across your feet, with heels firmly planted on the ground.

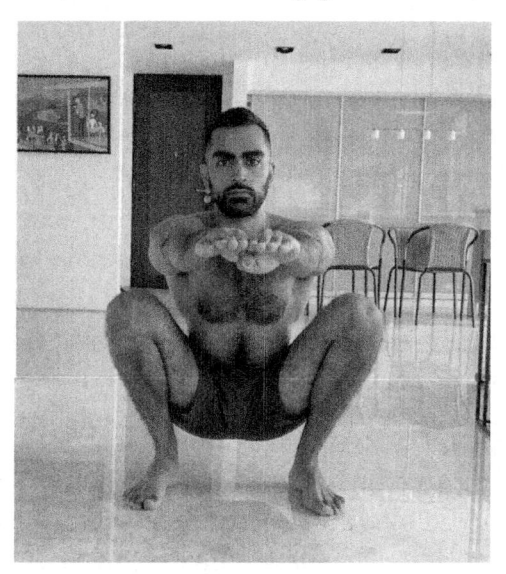

- Follow-through:
    1. As you enter into the deep squat position, you can extend your arms in front of you for counterbalance.
    2. Breathe deeply, allowing your hips to open and your spine to decompress.
    3. Keep your heels grounded, chest upright, and core lightly engaged.
    4. Hold for 30-60 seconds.

For those who struggle with this position, the deep squat hold provides an accessible pathway back to mobility. Start by holding onto a stable surface, such as a doorframe or counter, to ease into the posture. Gradually increase your time in the squat, focusing on deep breathing and relaxing into the stretch. With consistent practice, you can regain the full range of motion your body was designed to achieve, reclaiming the fluidity and freedom of movement that many of us lose with age and inactivity.

Horse Stance

The horse stance, a staple in various Eastern martial arts, is a powerful posture that symbolizes strength, stability, and endurance. With feet positioned wider than shoulder-width apart, knees bent, and hips lowered, the horse stance is much more than a static exercise—it's a dynamic way to build lower body strength, enhance hip mobility, and develop core stability. This posture demands your body to maintain balance and control in a deeply engaged position, making it a fundamental tool for cultivating resilience and mobility in the hips and spine.

In martial arts, practitioners are taught to root themselves to the ground, drawing strength from the earth while maintaining an unwavering base. This requires intense activation of the quads, glutes, and hip adductors, as well as strong engagement of the core muscles to stabilize the pelvis and support the spine. The lower you sink into the horse stance, the more these muscles are challenged to sustain the position, building both muscular endurance and mental focus.

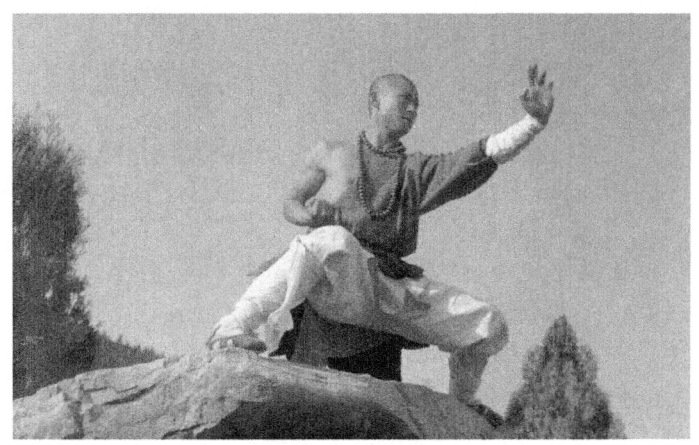

Known as "Ma Bu" in China, the horse stance has been a staple of Eastern martial arts styles for centuries. Holding this posture for extended periods of time is a means of developing focus in the mind and strength in the legs, providing martial artists with a stable foundation and strong legs for kicking techniques.

From an anatomical perspective, the horse stance offers a wide range of benefits. By lowering the hips and bending the knees, you stretch and strengthen the inner thigh muscles (adductors) while simultaneously improving hip mobility. This increased mobility facilitates everyday movements with greater ease and also helps prevent injuries by ensuring that your hips move freely through a wider range of motion. The stance also promotes an upright posture, which aligns the spine and engages the core, providing protection to the lower back by reducing strain and encouraging spinal stability.

Beyond mobility, the horse stance also plays a role in developing lower body power. Holding this position isometrically activates the fast-twitch muscle fibers, which are essential for explosive movements such as jumping, sprinting, and kicking. By strengthening these fibers, you enhance your ability to generate force quickly and efficiently, a critical aspect of athletic performance. In this way, the horse stance bridges the gap between static strength and dynamic power, preparing the body for more complex and demanding movements.

Steps to Perform the Horse Stance:

- Setup:
    1. Stand with your feet wider than shoulder-width apart, typically about 1.5 to 2 times your shoulder width.
    2. Your toes can point slightly outward (approximately 15-30 degrees), depending on your hip mobility and comfort.

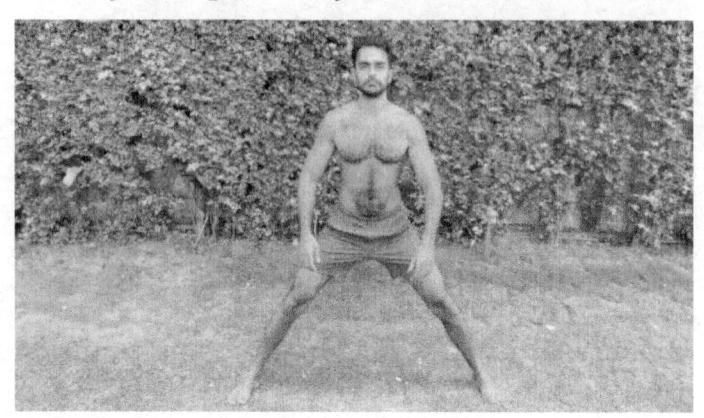

- Execution:
    1. Begin by bending your knees and lowering your hips directly down toward the ground, as though you're sitting into an invisible chair.
    2. Your thighs should move towards a parallel position with the floor, and your knees should track in the same direction as your toes.

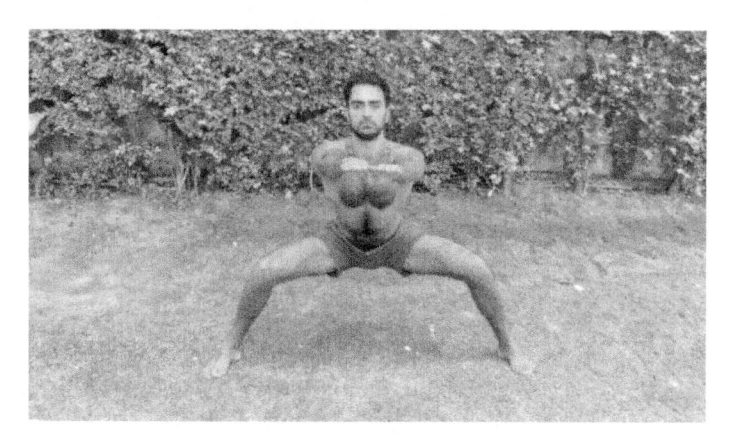

- Follow-through:
    1. Keep your weight evenly distributed across your feet, pressing firmly through both heels and the balls of your feet for balance.
    2. Maintain an upright posture with your spine in a neutral position—avoid rounding your lower back or leaning too far forward.
    3. Your head should remain in line with your spine and your gaze should be forward.
    4. Keep breathing deeply, focusing on relaxing into the stretch while holding tension in the muscles.

In Eastern practices, the horse stance is considered a meditative posture because holding it for extended periods requires both physical strength and mental fortitude. You must remain focused and present, overcoming discomfort to maintain the position, which sharpens your concentration and resilience. This mental toughness complements the physical strength gained, making the horse stance a powerful exercise for both body and mind.

Whether you're training for martial arts, looking to enhance your athleticism, or simply aiming to improve lower body strength and mobility, the horse stance is a valuable tool that connects the power of your lower body with the stability of your core and alignment of your spine. It is a dynamic exercise that reinforces both physical capability and mental resilience, forming a crucial component of any well-rounded training regimen.

Posterior To Anterior Pelvic Tilt

Practicing this movement develops greater awareness and control of your pelvic positioning—which is crucial for proper core engagement and spinal protection. In this exercise, performed in an elbow plank position, you actively tilt your pelvis between posterior and anterior positions. This controlled movement teaches you to recognize and adjust your pelvic tilt, a skill that many people lack, which often leads to poor posture, lack of core engagement, and an increased risk of spinal strain or injury.

Steps to Perform Posterior to Anterior Pelvic Tilt:

- Setup:
    1. Enter into an elbow plank position and engage your pelvis into posterior tilt, i.e. contract your glutes and engage your lower abdominals, pulling your pubic bone toward your ribcage.

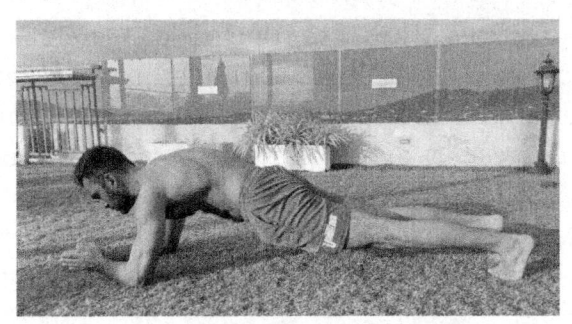

- Execution:
    1. Next, slowly transition into an anterior pelvic tilt by allowing your pelvis to tilt forward, arching your lower back slightly.
    2. In this position, you will feel your hip flexors

lengthening, and your core will disengage slightly as your pelvis shifts forward.

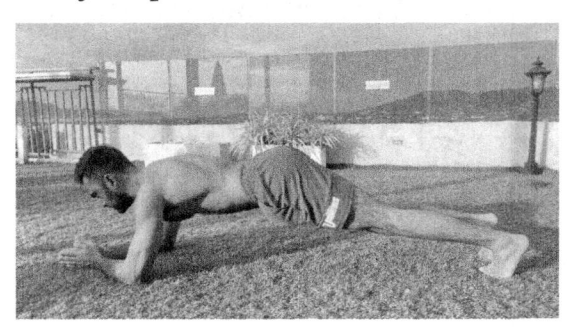

- Follow-through:
    1. Continue to alternate between the posterior and anterior pelvic tilts in a slow, controlled manner.
    2. Focus on feeling the movement in your pelvis and lower spine, and avoid excessive movement in your upper body or hips.

The pelvis acts as the body's central bridge, connecting the spine to the hips. Any misalignment in the pelvis, whether too far forward (anterior tilt) or tucked too far under (posterior tilt), disrupts the balance of the entire kinetic chain. When people lack proprioceptive awareness of their pelvic position, they are unable to properly engage their core muscles, leaving the spine vulnerable to bearing loads it wasn't designed to handle. Over time, this can contribute to issues such as lower back pain, spinal damage, or injury, especially during dynamic movements like lifting, running, or jumping.

The movement from posterior to anterior pelvic tilt is crucial because it helps you develop mind-muscle connection. When done correctly, the exercise teaches you how to engage and release your core muscles at will, allowing you to find a neutral pelvis—where the core is optimally engaged and the spine is supported. This awareness improves your ability to stabilize the spine during athletic and everyday activities while promoting better mobility in the hips and pelvis.

Proper pelvic control plays a vital role in maintaining overall spinal health and posture. Without the ability to effectively manage pelvic tilt, the hips and spine become rigid, and compensatory patterns develop. By practicing this exercise, you can retrain your body to maintain better alignment and core engagement, protecting your spine from unnecessary strain and allowing for more fluid, efficient movement in both the hips and spine.

Arch Up

The arch up, performed in a prone position, is a movement that engages the muscles of your posterior chain, including the lower back, glutes, and hamstrings. By lifting both your arms and legs up off the floor, you activate muscles along your spine, particularly in the lumbar region, and strengthen the glutes, which are often weakened or neglected in modern lifestyles dominated by sitting. This exercise plays a key role in improving posture, spinal mobility, and overall balance in the body by restoring the natural strength and function of the posterior chain.

Steps to Perform the Arch Up:

- Setup:
    1. Start by lying face down (prone) on the floor with your legs extended straight behind you and your arms extended straight in front of you, forming a straight line from fingers to toes.
    2. Keep your head in a neutral position, with your forehead or chin gently resting on the ground, and your gaze toward the floor. Your arms and legs should remain relaxed as you prepare for the movement.

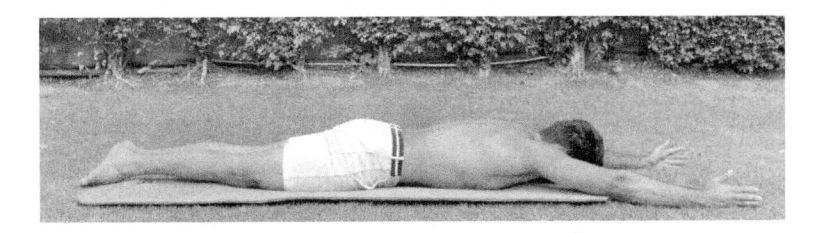

- Execution:
    1. Simultaneously lift your arms, chest, and legs up off the ground as high as you can.
    2. Focus on squeezing your glutes and engaging your lower back muscles to create the lift. Keep your chin tucked towards your chest.
    3. Your goal is to form an arch with your body, lifting as much of your torso and thighs up off the ground as you can.

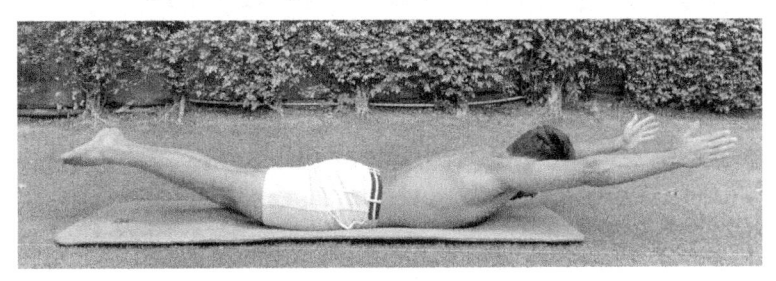

- Follow-through:
    1. You can choose to either perform repetitions or a static hold for a longer duration (e.g., 20-30 seconds or more), focusing on maintaining engagement in the lower back, glutes, and hamstrings.

When performing the arch up, you work the muscles that run along the spine, which serve to maintain alignment and protect the back from injury. These muscles, particularly the erector spinae, are responsible for keeping the spine extended and support the natural curvature of the lumbar region. Many people experience lower back pain due to weak lumbar muscles, leading to compensatory movements and poor posture. The arch up helps correct these imbalances by directly targeting the lumbar region and strengthening the entire back.

In addition to strengthening the lower back, the arch up also engages the glutes, which are often underused and weakened from long hours of sitting. The glutes are essential for stabilizing the pelvis and maintaining hip alignment. When the glutes are inactive or weak, it can lead to compromised movement patterns which increase strain on the lower back. By practicing the arch up, you can reawaken your gluteal muscles, enhancing hip mobility and stability, which in turn helps protect the spine from taking on excessive load.

Furthermore, the arch up encourages greater mobility in the hips and spine by counteracting the forward-leaning posture many people adopt in daily life. When you lift your arms and legs off the ground, you open up the front of your body and allow your spine to extend fully, promoting better range of motion in your back and hips. This movement helps restore balance between the anterior and posterior chains, ensuring that your body remains mobile from both sides.

Side Plank

The lateral chain of the body, which includes the muscles on the side of your torso, is often overlooked. The side plank is an excellent exercise for strengthening this area, particularly the obliques, which are crucial for rotational movements.

Steps to Perform a Side Plank:

- Setup:
    1. Begin by lying on your side with your legs extended and stacked on top of each other.
    2. Position your elbow directly under your shoulder, ensuring your forearm is flat on the ground and your upper arm is perpendicular to the floor.
    3. Engage your core by pulling your belly button

toward your spine, preparing to lift your body.
4. Keep your body in a straight line from your head to your heels, ensuring that your hips are not sagging or raised too high.

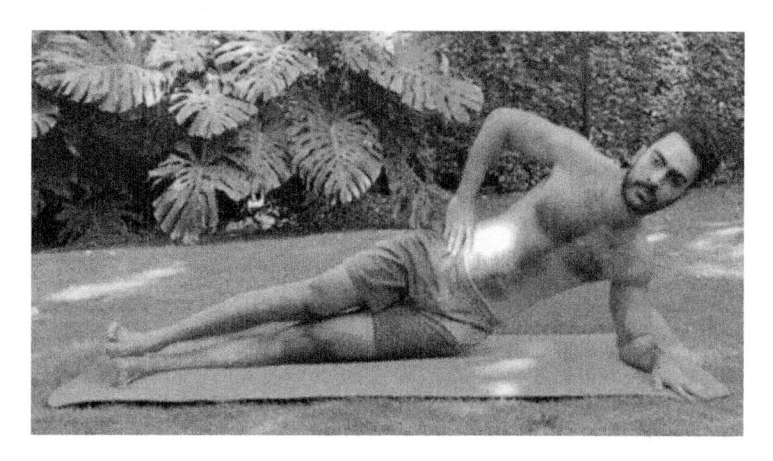

- Execution:
    1. Press down through your elbow and the edge of your bottom foot to lift your hips off the floor.
    2. Hold this position, making sure your body forms a straight line from your head to your feet.
    3. Keep your head in line with your spine, and gaze forward or slightly down for neck alignment.
    4. Engage your glutes and core throughout the movement to maintain stability.

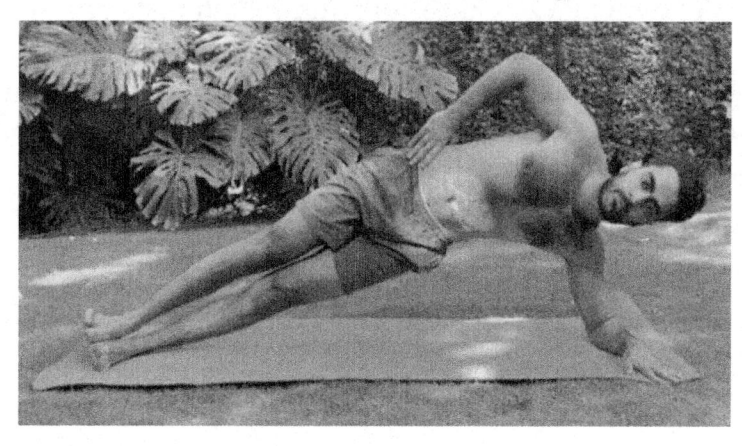

- Follow-through:
    1. You can hold the position for the desired amount of time (e.g., 30-60 seconds) or perform reps.
    2. To release, slowly lower your hips back to the ground in a controlled manner.
    3. Rest for a few seconds, then switch sides to repeat on the other side.

Each of the above exercises targets key muscle groups and joints that are often neglected in modern life. When practiced consistently, they not only enhance mobility but also restore natural movement patterns that protect you from pain and injury.

By prioritizing the mobility of your hips and spine, you're investing in your body's long-term functionality. As you continue with these movements, you'll notice improved posture, reduced stiffness, and a newfound fluidity in your everyday life. Remember, mobility is about freedom of movement, ensuring that your body remains agile and pain-free for years to come.

Programming For The Hips & Spine

We will dive deep on how to program your workouts in Chapter 11, which will allow you to mix and match different exercises into a routine that fits your situation. The following workout is provided as an example. You can follow it as is, observe how you feel, and figure out what areas of your body require more of your focus.

Sample Hips & Spine Mobility Workout

1. Deep squat hold: 1 set x 30-60 second hold
2. Horse stance hold: 1 set x 30-60 second hold

> 3. Posterior to anterior pelvic tilt: 3 sets x 10-15 reps
>
> *Perform exercises 3-5 in a circuit, i.e. one after the other with 1-3 minutes rest between rounds.*
>
> 4. Arch up: 3 sets x 10-15 reps
>
> 5. Side plank: 3 sets x 10-15 reps

Mobility Matters Most

Throughout this chapter, we explored how proper alignment distributes stress evenly across your body, allowing your joints, muscles, and connective tissues to function harmoniously. By building mobility from the ground up—starting with your feet, ankles, and knees—you create a resilient foundation that stays protected against injury.

In the opening story, we saw how my lack of awareness around alignment led to repeated knee injuries. Like a building with a faulty foundation, my body crumbled under pressure. But through the discovery of mobility training, I learned that strength alone is not enough; the joints must be able to move through a wide range of motion.

In the next chapter, I'll share mobility exercises specifically for the upper body. You'll discover how seemingly minor restrictions can have a cascading effect, setting the stage for chronic issues and injuries. You'll get a roadmap to addressing these areas, equipping you with the tools to maintain a balanced, pain-free body that can meet the demands of your training and daily life.

Ultimately, the key to long-term fitness success is cultivating a body that remains aligned and moves effortlessly, so you can push your limits without fear of injury. Turn to the next page as we continue to address the root causes of pain and discomfort, helping you build a resilient and capable body from the ground up.

Chapter Takeaways

• Alignment isn't just about posture; it's about ensuring that your body moves efficiently. When your joints are aligned, they distribute force properly, preventing compensations that lead to pain and injury.

• The greater control you have over a wider range of motion, the more resilient your joints will be against the pressures of training and daily life. Mobility training can work for rehabilitation and it's also a proactive approach for building a body that can withstand physical stresses.

• Prioritizing lower body mobility ensures that the foundational elements of your movement are strong and stable. A focus on feet, ankles, and knees prepares your body to handle forces effectively, creating a stable base for upper body activities.

• Ignoring mobility in key areas forces other parts of your body to compensate, leading to a chain reaction of dysfunction. Painful conditions like plantar fasciitis, knee pain, and lower back issues often have roots in poor alignment and limited mobility in seemingly unrelated areas.

• Incorporating movements like backward walking, tibialis raises, and FHL calf raises can dramatically improve lower leg function and protect your knees. Similarly, exercises targeting the hips and spine, like the deep squat hold and horse stance, enhance overall stability and range of motion, reducing the risk of injury.

FREE GOODWILL

"The greatest gift you can give another is a pathway to their own potential."

—UNKNOWN

By this point in the book, you've already taken the first steps toward building a stronger, more capable body—and I hope you're finding real value in the journey so far. But before we dive deeper, I have a small favor to ask.

We live in a world where our choices are often influenced by what others say. A single review can make the difference between someone discovering the life-changing potential of calisthenics or missing out entirely. So here's where you can help.

If this book has been helpful to you so far, would you take a moment to leave a quick, honest review? It'll take less than 60 seconds, costs nothing, and could be the nudge someone else needs to start their own journey.

Your review could be the reason someone:

- Decides to heal their body instead of enduring more pain
- Finds the courage to take control of their health and well-being

- Learns how to move better, feel better, and live better

To leave a review:

- On Kindle or an e-reader, scroll to the bottom and swipe up to be prompted for a review.
- On Amazon, simply head to the book's page and leave your thoughts along with a star rating.
- On audible, hit the three dots in the upper right corner of your screen, click rate & review, then leave a few sentences about your view on the book along with a star rating.

I'm not asking for praise—just your honest take. If there's something you liked (or didn't), I want to know, and so do others.

Your voice matters. You've already taken action by getting to this point of the book, and this is a way to share that value with others. Your support means the world to me, and together, we can help more people move toward health, strength, and lasting vitality.

Thank you for your time, your energy, and for being part of this journey.

Now, let's get back to work on mastering the body you were designed to move in.

CHAPTER 8 - CREATING ALIGNMENT PART II

"Training is something you will be doing your whole life. When you see it that way then you won't be in a rush. The best gains are made over long periods of time."

—NICOLAS DE PAOLI

He was determined.

After years of failed attempts, my client, we'll call him Michael, had still not given up on his goal of unlocking his first pull up.

"I've been trying for years," he told me, frustration etched on his face. For the past few months, he'd been pushing himself harder than ever, convinced that sheer force of will would finally get his chin over the bar. But instead of the victory he craved, Michael found himself wrestling with a different reality: sharp, persistent pain shooting through his right elbow every time he tried to pull himself up.

When I watched him train, the problem was immediately clear. Michael's approach was all wrong. He was relying almost entirely on his arms, neglecting to engage his back, and ignoring the crucial role his shoulder blades needed to play. His elbows, the weakest link in this faulty chain, were bearing the brunt of his efforts. I could see it—his backside was completely uninvolved, his shoulders hunched forward, and his movements were all over the place, desperately compensating for what was missing: control, alignment, and mobility.

Michael's story is far from unique. In a hurry to master exercises like pull ups and push ups, many people rush the process, thinking they're working on a simple exercise, only to find that they're actually setting themselves back. This isn't just about effort; it's about understanding the hidden complexities of movement and knowing the progression that allows you to build strength without sacrificing your joints. The truth is, your upper body's ability to move efficiently hinges on one critical element that's often overlooked—scapula mobility.

The scapula (aka shoulder blades) is the linchpin of your upper body because there isn't a single upper body movement that doesn't involve this essential structure. When it's functioning well, your scapula allows your arms and shoulders to move freely through different planes of motion. But without proper mobility and control, compensations occur, often leading to pain in the shoulders, elbows, or wrists. Just as a misaligned foundation can destabilize an entire building, dysfunction in the scapula ripples outward, compromising your upper body strength, performance, and joint health.

In this chapter, we'll explore why scapular mobility is the cornerstone of effective upper body movement. We'll discuss the critical roles the scapula plays, the common mistakes that lead to compensations, and the exercises that will help you mobilize, strengthen, and stabilize this vital area. We'll also extend our focus to the shoulders, elbows, and wrists—key joints that, when properly mobilized, work synergistically with the scapula to create a resilient upper body.

By the end of this chapter, you'll understand that there's far more to exercises like pull ups and push ups than meets the eye. You'll learn how to avoid the pitfalls of compensatory patterns and gain the tools needed to unlock pain-free movement, not just during exercise, but in every aspect of your life. Because when your scapula is mobile, your entire upper body thrives.

Scapula Engagement: The Key To Structural Balance

The scapula is more than just a bone that sits on your back; it's a dynamic, mobile structure that supports upper body movement in general. Acting as a bridge between your arms and spine, the scapula is essential for transferring force and providing stability during pushing, pulling, lifting, and rotating actions. Yet, despite its importance, the scapula is often overlooked in traditional training, leading to imbalances that can set you up for pain and injury.

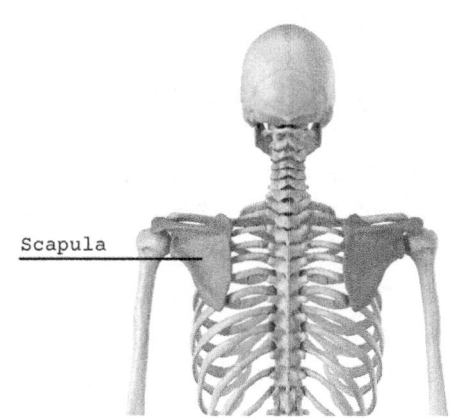

Positioned on the back of your ribcage, the scapula acts as the central hub connecting your arms to your spine. It's like a bridge that transfers force between your upper body and the rest of your

body, allowing you to generate power and move efficiently.

Proper alignment and mobility in the muscles surrounding the scapula ensure smooth coordination between the shoulder blades and arms, reducing the risk of impingement or overuse injuries. In addition to facilitating upper body movement, the scapula plays a key role in maintaining proper posture. When the scapula is retracted and depressed—pulled back and down—it helps open the chest and align the spine, counteracting the forward-leaning posture many people develop from prolonged sitting or desk work. This positioning encourages better alignment of the head, neck, and spine, reducing strain on the upper back while promoting more efficient movement.

In contrast, poor scapular mobility can lead to rounded shoulders and a hunched posture, placing undue stress on the neck and upper back. Over time, these postural imbalances can lead to chronic discomfort or injury. Developing awareness of scapular positioning and control is essential for preventing these issues and ensuring that the upper body remains strong, mobile, and resilient.

◆ ◆ ◆

Charles Poloquin was a highly respected strength coach and exercise scientist in the 90s and 2000s who was known for his ability to get elite athletes back to full functionality after severe injuries. He developed the Structural Balance Theory that emphasizes the importance of achieving balance between opposing muscle groups to ensure that your body functions efficiently and remains injury free. This concept is especially critical when it comes to the scapula.

As a coach, I've consistently observed my clients to have stronger anterior muscles—like the chest, biceps, and front deltoids—compared to their posterior muscles, particularly those that support and control the scapula. This imbalance often stems from focusing too much on the muscles we see in the mirror and neglecting the less visible but equally important muscles on the back of the body. The result is a structural imbalance that compensates for these weaknesses, leading to common issues like rounded shoulders, shoulder impingement, and chronic upper back or neck pain. Many people mistakenly think their shoulder problems are caused by the shoulder joint itself, but the root cause often lies in the imbalance between the overdeveloped anterior muscles and the underdeveloped posterior chain.

Proper scapula engagement is how you activate your posterior chain. When the scapula is mobile, it allows the back muscles to activate and support the shoulders, creating a balanced and powerful upper body. The beauty of calisthenics is that it naturally encourages total body engagement. When performed correctly, many calisthenics exercises require not just brute strength but also control, coordination, and stability throughout the entire body. Yet, without proper scapular mobility, this total engagement remains out of reach, and people end up stuck, unable to progress and prone to injury.

In this chapter, we'll dive into specific exercises that build scapula mobility, stability, and control. Whether you're doing pull ups, push ups, or advanced calisthenics, these movements are stepping stones that allow you to engage the right muscles at the right time, ensuring you can progress safely and effectively.

Mobility Exercises For The Scapula

The scapula moves in four key directions—protraction, retraction, elevation, and depression—all of which are essential for balanced upper body movement.

Protraction involves moving the shoulder blades apart and away from the spine, while retraction brings the shoulder blades together toward the spine. Depression lowers the shoulder blades down and away from the ears while elevation lifts them up toward the ears. Mastering these four movements is fundamental. Without proper scapular control, the surrounding muscles and joints are forced to bear loads they are not designed to handle, leading to poor posture and increased injury risk.

By practicing the following exercises, you'll develop the mind-muscle connection necessary to engage your scapula. Mobilizing the scapula also protects your shoulders, arms, and back by ensuring that your body moves efficiently without compensation. Whether you're new to training or looking to refine your technique, these exercises will set you up for long-term success in your calisthenics journey.

Scapula Push Up

The scapula push up is a deceptively simple exercise that serves as a prerequisite for proper push up technique. In a scapula push up, you remain in a push up position with your elbows locked, but instead of bending your arms, the movement comes exclusively from your scapula, cycling between active scapular protraction (pushing the shoulder blades apart) and passive scapular retraction (squeezing them together).

Steps to Perform a Scapula Push Up:

- Setup:
    1. Start in a push up position with your hands placed shoulder-width apart on the floor, directly underneath your shoulders. Keep your legs extended and your toes pressing into the floor.
    2. Activate your glutes, quads, and core to maintain stability in your body. Your neck should remain neutral, with your gaze slightly forward.
    3. Protract your scapula, pushing through your hands and separating your shoulder blades as far apart as possible. This will cause your upper back

to round slightly as your chest moves away from the floor.

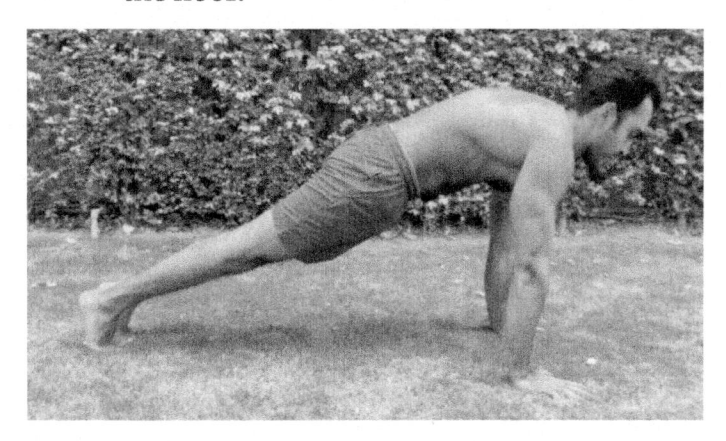

- Execution:
    1. Get into scapular retraction by bringing your shoulder blades together, squeezing them toward your spine as your chest lowers slightly toward the floor. Remember to keep your elbows locked, isolating the movement in the scapula rather than bending the arms.

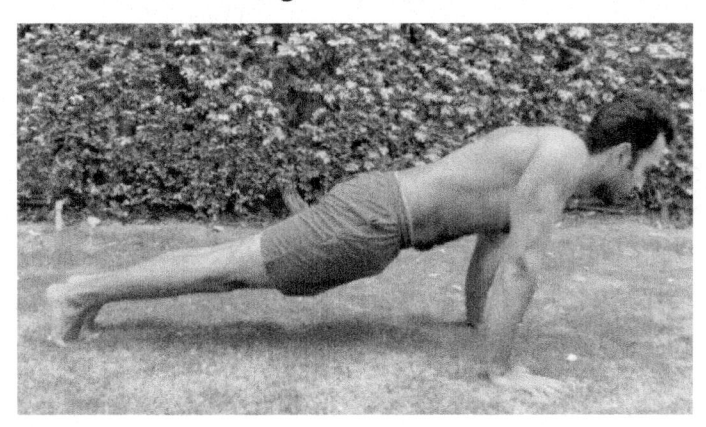

- Follow-through:
    1. Continue cycling between these two positions, smoothly moving from active protraction to passive retraction.
    2. Ensure each phase of the movement is slow

and controlled, focusing on scapular engagement rather than speed or intensity.

Although it seems basic, this exercise is a game-changer for anyone looking to perform push ups correctly and avoid common issues that arise from poor form. Most people skip this foundational step, resulting in faulty push up technique that can lead to wrist, elbow, and shoulder issues over time. Without proper scapular engagement, the body compensates by placing too much strain on smaller joints and muscles, leading to imbalances and discomfort.

In gymnastics, this movement is taught early, but many of us missed that lesson, and as a result, we push up incorrectly —failing to engage the scapula and the posterior chain. The scapula push up teaches you to recruit the lats and the larger muscles of the back by focusing on scapular protraction, which helps balance the load across your entire upper body, ensuring that the movement is more efficient and that the scapula can support the shoulders properly. Without mastering the scapula push up, most people never experience the push up as a total-body exercise.

By practicing scapula push ups, you'll not only build scapular strength and mobility but also prepare your body for more advanced movements. Mastering this movement will improve your overall body awareness and bring your push up technique to the next level.

Rear Scapula Push Up

The rear scapula push up offers a unique variation that targets the scapula from a different angle, reinforcing control and strength. While the standard scapula push up focuses on active protraction and passive retraction, the rear scapula push up emphasizes active retraction and passive protraction. By changing your orientation—where your back is facing the ground rather than your chest—you adjust the pull of gravity, allowing you to engage and work the scapular muscles from a different perspective.

Steps to Perform a Rear Scapula Push Up:

- Setup:
    1. Start by sitting on the ground with your feet flat and knees bent. Place your hands on the ground behind you, shoulder-width apart, with your fingers pointing either in the opposite direction of your feet or at a slight angle, depending on your wrist comfort.

- Execution:
    1. Lift your hips up off the ground so that your body is supported by your hands and feet, similar to a reverse tabletop position. Keep your arms straight, locking your elbows out, and engage your core and glutes to maintain stability.
    2. Ensure that your shoulders are above your wrists, and your body forms a straight line from your shoulders to your knees, avoiding sagging in the hips.
    3. Retract your scapula—squeeze your shoulder blades together, allowing your chest to puff upward as your upper back engages.

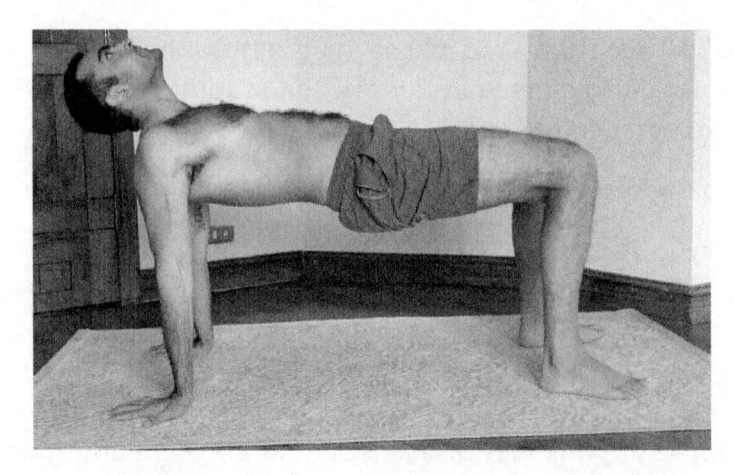

- Follow-through:
    1. Enter scapula protraction by allowing your shoulder blades to spread apart passively, as your chest lowers slightly and your upper back rounds. Keep your elbows locked and your glutes engaged to ensure that the movement comes from your scapula and not from bending your arms or lower body.

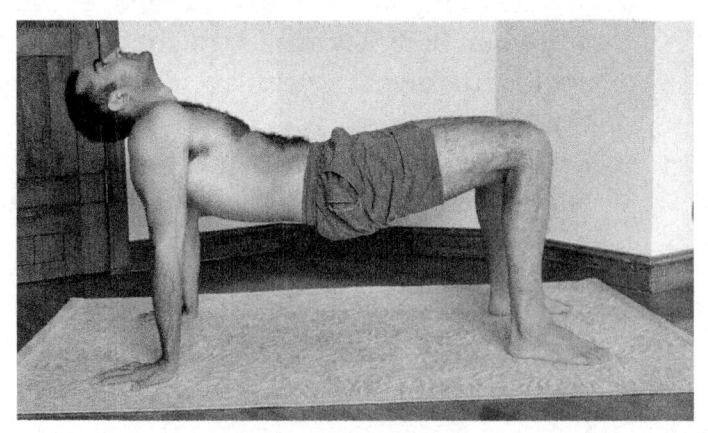

While the standard scapula push up teaches you to control the forward movement of your shoulder blades, the rear scapula push up enhances your ability to retract them, which is vital for pulling exercises like rows and pull ups. Additionally, proper scapular retraction supports good posture by preventing the shoulders from rounding forward.

Many people lack strength and control in scapular retraction, which can lead to imbalances and compensatory patterns, particularly in pulling exercises. The rear scapula push up helps correct this by isolating the scapula's retraction and protraction in a controlled environment, ensuring that the shoulders and upper back are engaged correctly. By mastering both active protraction (scapula push up) and active retraction (rear scapula push up), you develop structural balance in the scapula.

Practicing the rear scapula push up helps reinforce scapular stability, improve posture, and strengthen the muscles that support shoulder and upper back mobility. This exercise ensures that your scapula is fully engaged in both pushing and pulling movements, giving you a solid foundation for more advanced exercises and creating balance in the musculature of your upper body.

Seated Scapula Lift

This exercise develops scapular mobility and control for vertical pushing movements like dips where you need to stabilize the shoulders by keeping the scapula down and away from the ears. In this movement, you sit with your legs extended in front of you, and through scapular depression, you press your hands into the floor, lifting your hips off the ground. Conversely, allowing your hips to lower back down as your shoulders rise into passive scapular elevation helps you understand how to control the movement without compensating with elbow bend or upper arm tension.

Steps to Perform a Seated Scapula Lift:

- Setup:
    1. Sit on the floor with your legs extended out in front of you, keeping your feet together and your knees fully locked. Place your hands on yoga

blocks next to your hips
2. Actively depress your scapula by pressing your hands into the yoga blocks so that your shoulders pull down and away from your ears as your hips lift up off the floor.

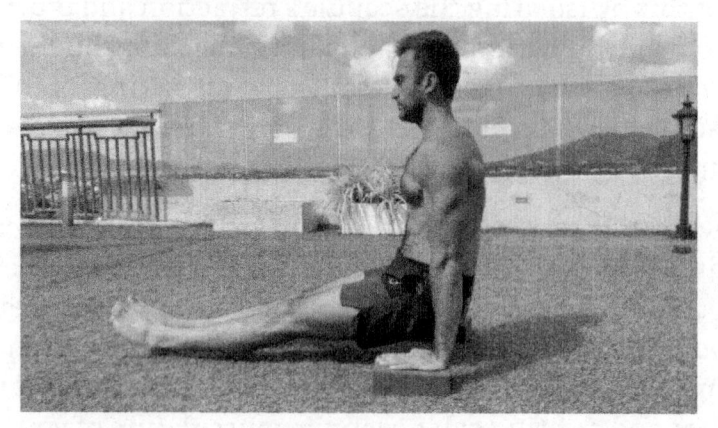

- Execution:
    1. Hold the lifted position for 1-2 seconds, feeling the engagement in your shoulders, lats, and upper back. This is the active scapular depression phase.
    2. Slowly allow your hips to lower back toward the floor as your shoulders rise up toward your ears (passive scapular elevation). Ensure that your elbows stay locked, focusing on the controlled upward movement of the scapula.

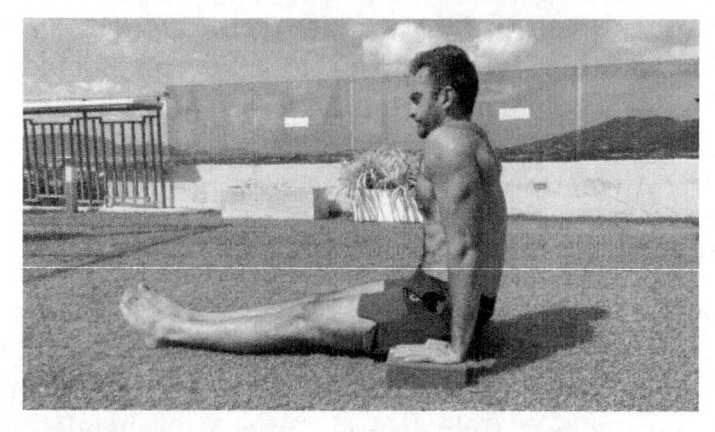

- Follow-through:
    1. Continue alternating between active scapular depression (lifting your hips) and passive scapular elevation (lowering your hips). Focus on isolating the movement to the scapula and avoid using your arms or upper traps to compensate.
    2. As you progress and gain more control over the scapula, aim to increase your hold time in the active depression phase or try performing the exercise without blocks for added difficulty.

Practicing this exercise lays the groundwork for performing vertical pushing movements with greater strength, mobility, and stability in your scapula.

Scapula Pull Up

This exercise focuses on the movement from passive scapular elevation (where the shoulders are up toward the ears) to active scapular depression (where the shoulders are pulled down away from the ears). This movement is the opposite of the seated scapula lift, and it is essential for mastering exercises like pull ups and chin ups. Many people, even those capable of performing full pull ups, lack the scapular control necessary to fully engage their upper back muscles, often relying too heavily on their arms to initiate the movement. This over-reliance can lead to compensatory patterns, particularly in the elbows, and may contribute to common issues like elbow pain or shoulder strain.

Steps to Perform a Scapula Pull Up:

- Setup:
    1. Begin by gripping a bar with your hands slightly wider than shoulder-width apart, palms facing forward (overhand grip). Hang from the bar with your arms fully extended and your feet off the ground, allowing your body to relax into a passive

hang where your shoulders elevate near your ears. Your body should be in a straight line, with your core engaged to maintain stability.

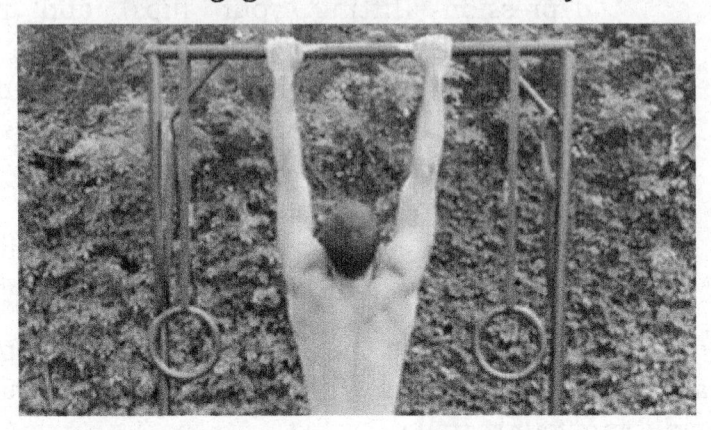

- Execution:
    1. From the passive hang, initiate the movement by actively depressing your scapula—pull your shoulder blades down and away from your ears. This action should cause your chest to rise slightly toward the bar as your shoulders move away from your ears, engaging the muscles in your upper back, specifically your lats and lower trapezius.
    2. Hold the active depression for 1-2 seconds, ensuring that the movement is controlled and that you feel the engagement in your upper back and shoulders.

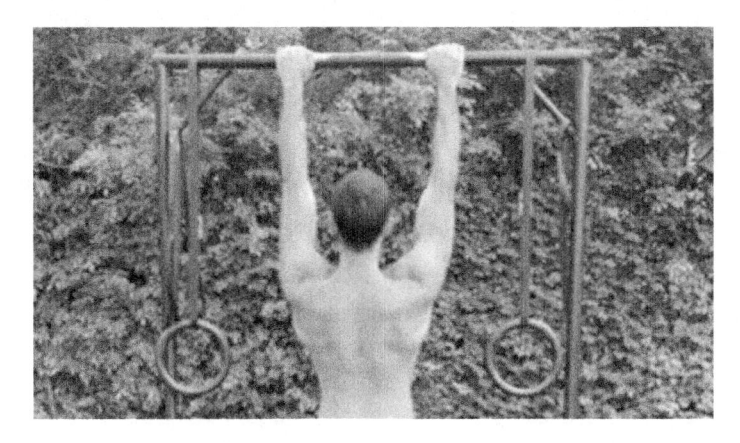

- Follow-through:
    1. Slowly return to the passive scapula elevation by allowing your shoulders to elevate toward your ears as you lower your chest slightly. Keep the movement smooth and controlled, resisting the urge to use your arms or elbows.
    2. Keep your elbows fully locked throughout the movement to isolate the scapula.
    3. As you progress, aim to increase the hold duration in the active depression phase and work toward greater control and range of motion. You can eventually incorporate this movement as part of your warm-up or integrate it into your pull up progression.

The scapula pull up teaches you how to initiate the pull up from your scapula, rather than your arms. By learning how to actively depress your scapula at the beginning of the movement, you recruit the larger muscles of your back, such as the lats and lower trapezius, to do the work, thus reducing strain on the smaller tissues and joints like the bicep tendon and elbows. This scapular awareness is critical not only for preventing injuries but also for maximizing the effectiveness of the pulling exercises, as it allows you to engage your entire upper body efficiently.

In a typical pull up, failure to properly depress the scapula at the start of the movement leads to an overuse of the arm muscles, which places unnecessary stress on the elbows and can lead to conditions like golfer's elbow (medial epicondylitis) or tennis elbow (lateral epicondylitis). Learning the scapula pull up corrects this by training you to initiate movement with the scapula and ensure the shoulders are stable and properly aligned before progressing to the full pull up.

Whether you're a beginner working toward your first pull up or someone looking to refine your technique, the scapula pull up is a vital exercise that ensures proper scapular engagement, building both strength and mobility. It paves the way for mastering pull ups with efficient movement, injury prevention, and posterior chain activation.

The above exercises may seem simple, but they're very powerful. When you do them, focus on how your shoulder blades are moving. It's not about going through the motions; it's about consciously controlling and feeling your scapula in action.

Scapula engagement is an often neglected aspect of correct exercise execution and injury avoidance. In my experience as a coach, I've observed one hundred percent of new clients struggle with proper technique on exercises as apparently simple as the push up because they aren't aware of how to properly engage their scapula. Long term, this can lead to pinched shoulders and flared elbows—a recipe for injury.

Understanding and controlling your scapula is about building a strong, mobile, and injury-proof upper body. By focusing on your scapula, you're taking the first step towards mastering proper exercise technique. Remember, it's about quality of movement, not quantity of reps. Start incorporating these exercises into your routine and feel the difference in your strength, mobility and stability across all upper body exercises.

Mobility Exercises For The Wrists, Elbows, & Shoulders

While the scapula serves as the linchpin of the upper body, it's important not to overlook the ancillary joints that support it. These joints bear significant loads during various movements, making their conditioning crucial for overall mobility and injury prevention.

The wrists, elbows, and shoulders are often subjected to repetitive stresses and strains, particularly in activities involving gripping, pushing, and lifting. Without adequate preparation and regular mobilization, these joints can become susceptible to overuse injuries, impingements, and chronic discomfort. Therefore, incorporating targeted mobility exercises into your routine is essential to fortify these areas, ensuring they remain resilient and functional.

In this section, we will dive into the exercises that enhance wrist, elbow, and shoulder mobility. By focusing on these joints, you will not only improve your performance in various physical activities but also build a foundation that supports long-term health and vitality.

Wrist Mobilization

The wrists bear a significant amount of load during all upper body exercises, making their mobility essential for injury-prevention. For instance, many people I've worked with experience wrist pain during push ups. The common reason is that while they have developed strong chest and arm muscles from using machines, dumbbells, and barbells, their wrists haven't kept up. This imbalance is what creates discomfort and can even lead to injuries, as the wrists are not prepared to handle the stress.

To avoid these issues, it's important to incorporate wrist mobilization exercises into your routine. These exercises will help you build strength and flexibility in your wrists, ensuring they can support the load during various movements. By doing so, you'll reduce the risk of pain and injuries, allowing you to perform exercises like push ups more effectively and safely.

The following mobilization exercises will help you prepare your wrists for the demands of upper body workouts, promoting overall joint health and enhancing your performance.

Wrist extension. This is the movement of bending your wrist backward, increasing the angle between your hand and your forearm. This position gently stretches and strengthens the muscles and tendons in your wrists and forearms.

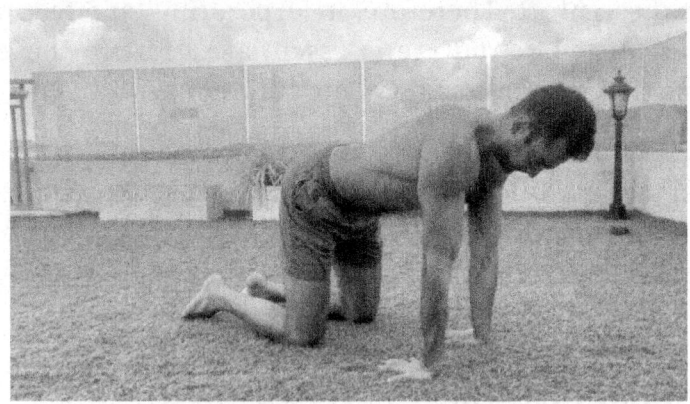

Start on your hands and knees with wrists under shoulders and fingers pointing back.

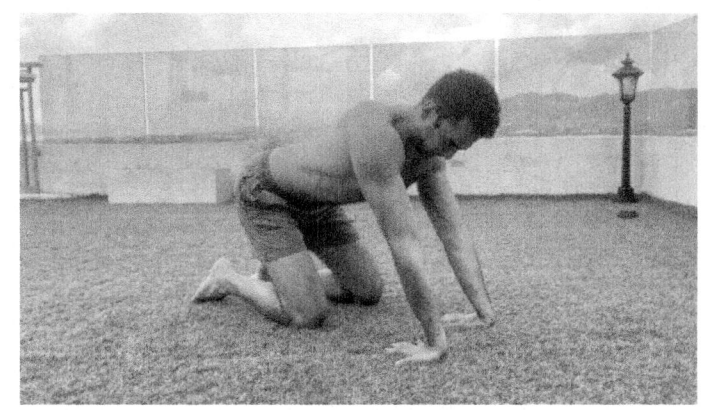

Then, lean back gently while keeping your palms planted on the floor to feel the stretch in your wrists and forearms. Return to the starting position and repeat for reps.

Wrist flexion. This is the movement of bending your wrist forward, decreasing the angle between your hand and your forearm.

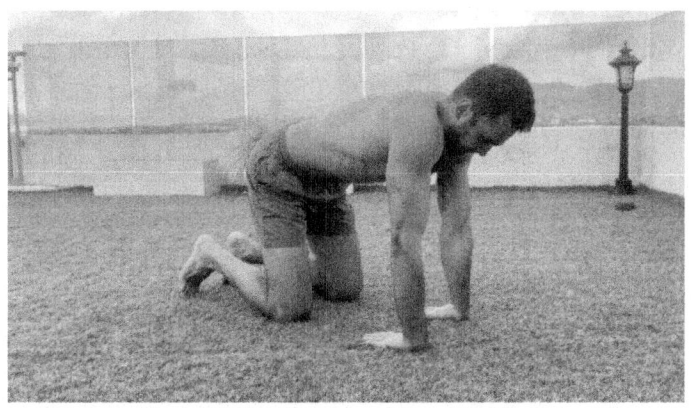

Start on your hands and knees with wrists under shoulders, but place the back of your hands on the floor with your fingers pointing back towards your knees.

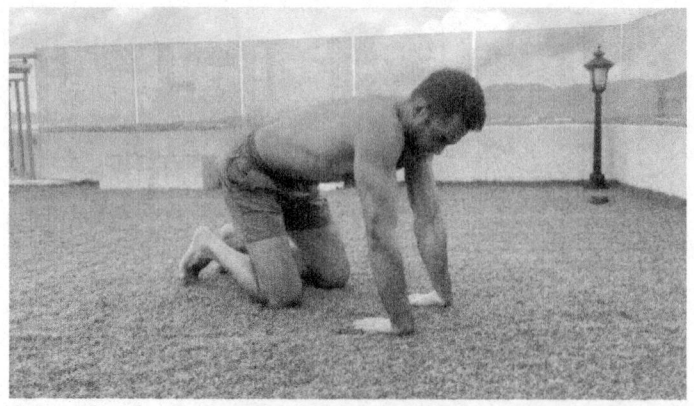

Then, slowly shift your body weight back towards your heels, feeling a stretch in your wrists and forearms. Return to the starting position and repeat for reps.

Wrist flexion and extension are vital for maintaining healthy and resilient wrists. These exercises help increase the mobility and strength of your wrist joints, preparing them to handle load during upper body movements. By taking the time to strengthen and mobilize your wrists, you create a solid foundation for your upper body, improving your overall performance and long-term joint health.

Remember, a balanced approach to training involves not only focusing on major muscle groups but also ensuring that the supporting joints and tendons are equally prepared. Prioritizing wrist health will enable you to perform a variety of exercises safely and effectively, leading to better results and a more enjoyable fitness journey.

Elbow Mobilization

Just like the wrists, the elbows are crucial joints that play a significant role in upper body movement. They are involved in almost every pushing and pulling exercise, bearing considerable loads and facilitating a wide range of motions. Without proper mobility, the elbows remain prone to injuries.

Many people overlook the importance of elbow health, focusing primarily on larger muscle groups. However, the elbows are essential for transferring force between the upper arm and forearm, making their strength and flexibility vital for effective and safe exercise execution.

The following exercises will help you prepare your elbows for the demands of upper body workouts, reducing the risk of pain and injury.

Straight elbow rotations. Practicing straight elbow rotations will improve elbow mobility and increase awareness of how your elbows can move through space. This exercise is performed in a quadruped position (on your hands and knees) and involves rotating your elbows through their full range of motion.

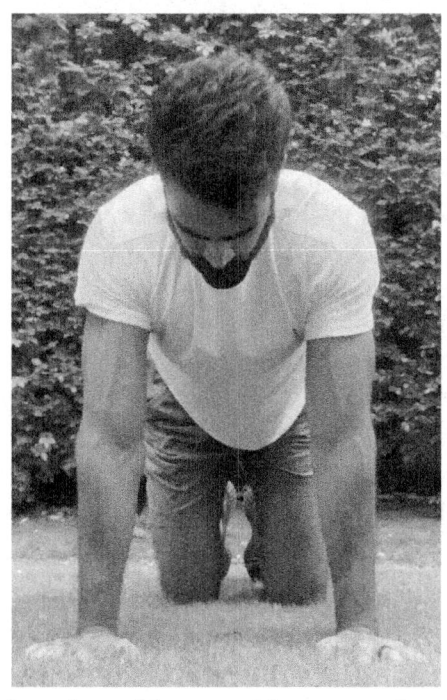

Start on your hands and knees with your wrists directly under your shoulders and your knees are under your hips.

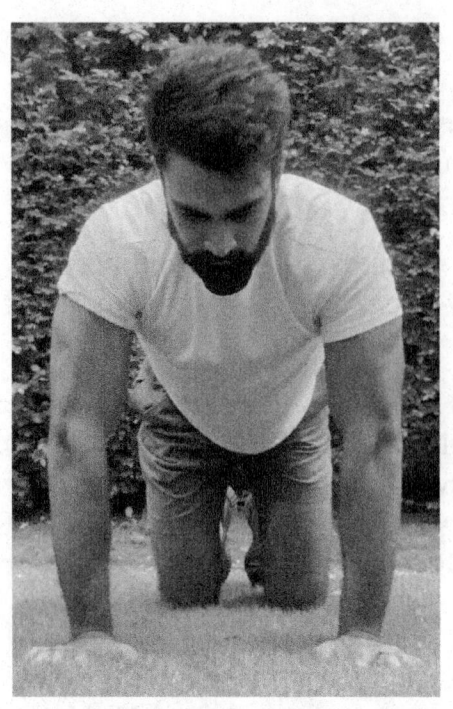

Rotate your elbows so that your elbow pits (the inner part of your elbows) point forward. This position externally rotates your elbows. Next, rotate your elbows in the opposite direction so that your elbows (the bony part) move towards forward. This position internally rotates your elbows.

Elbow push ups. This exercise is performed on all fours and involves lowering your body until your elbows touch the floor and then pushing back up. It's a simple movement that targets the muscles and tendons around the elbows, enhancing their stability and reducing the risk of injury during more demanding exercises.

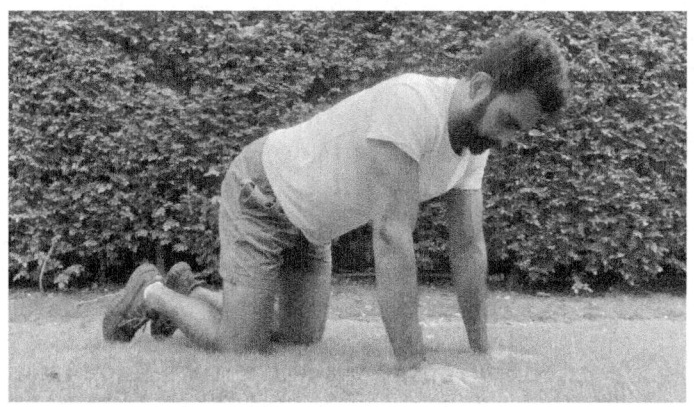

Start in a quadruped position on your hands and knees with wrists under shoulders and knees under hips.

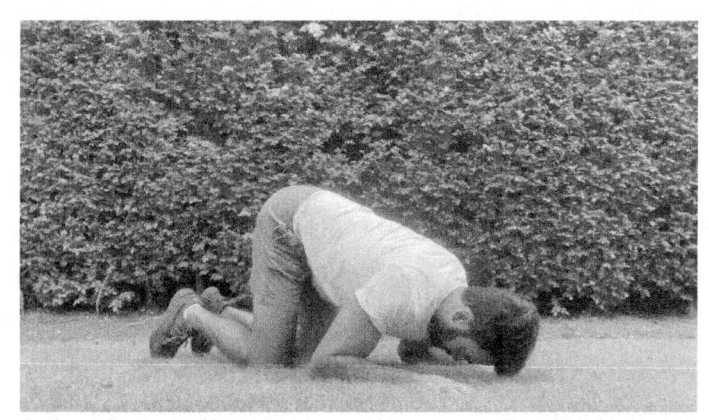

Slowly bend your elbows, lowering your upper body until your elbows touch the floor. From this position, press through your hands to straighten your arms, lifting your elbows off the floor and returning to the starting position. Repeat for reps.

The elbows are involved in nearly every pushing and pulling exercise, and without proper conditioning, they can become vulnerable to strains, overuse injuries, and discomfort. By paying attention to your elbow joints and incorporating targeted mobilization exercises like straight elbow rotations and elbow push ups, you can ensure that your elbows remain resilient.

Shoulder Mobilization

The shoulder, known as the glenohumeral, is the most mobile joint in the human body. It allows for a wide range of motion, enabling your arms to move in almost every direction. This incredible mobility is what makes the shoulder so vital for various movements, from lifting and throwing to pushing and pulling. However, this same mobility also makes the shoulder joint more susceptible to injury if it's not properly maintained.

It's important to differentiate the shoulder joint from the shoulder blades, or scapula. While the scapula plays a crucial role in stabilizing and guiding the movement of the shoulder, the shoulder joint itself requires its own attention. Many shoulder issues can often be traced back to limited mobility in the scapula, but the shoulder joint must also be capable of moving freely and efficiently through its full range of motion.

The following mobilization exercises are designed to enhance the mobility of your shoulder joint. By incorporating these exercises into your routine, you'll be taking important steps to protect your shoulders, improve your performance, and reduce the likelihood of injury.

Stick shoulder dislocates. This exercise involves using a stick, dowel, or resistance band to take your shoulders through a full range of motion, helping to open up the entire anterior side of the body. Practicing stick shoulder dislocates will help improve your shoulder joint's range of motion and prepare your shoulders for more demanding movements.

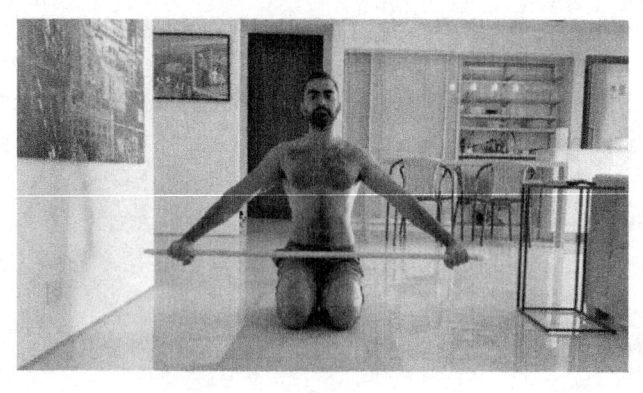

Start in a seated (or standing position) while holding a stick, dowel, or resistance band with both hands. Your grip should be wide enough to allow for smooth movement without discomfort.

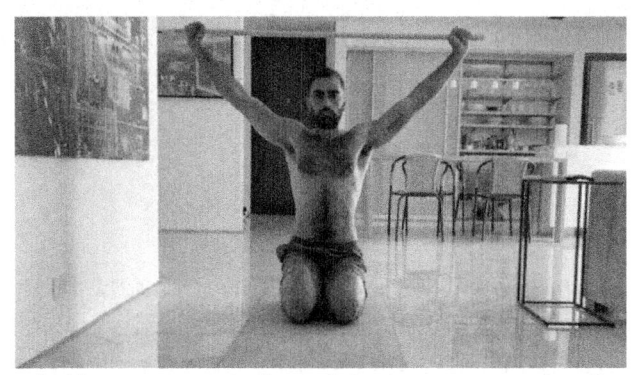

Begin the movement by raising your arms overhead while maintaining your grip on the stick or band.

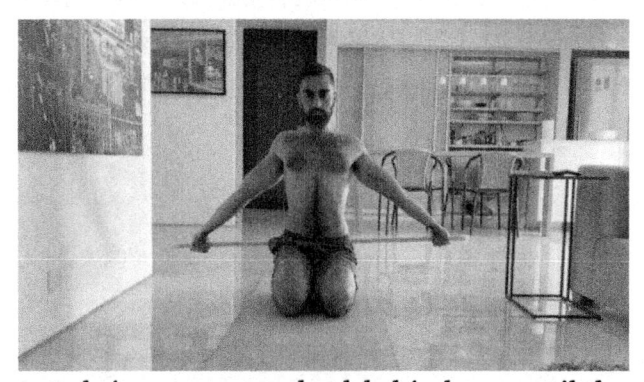

Continue to bring your arms back behind you until the stick or band reaches your lower back or buttocks. Slowly reverse the movement, bringing your arms back overhead and returning to the starting position in front of your body. Repeat for reps.

Stick shoulder extension. This is an excellent exercise for improving shoulder mobility, particularly in the posterior chain. This exercise involves standing in front of a wall with a stick or dowel held behind your back, focusing on extending your shoulders as far back as possible. It's a great way to open up the chest and shoulders while enhancing mobility in the shoulder joint.

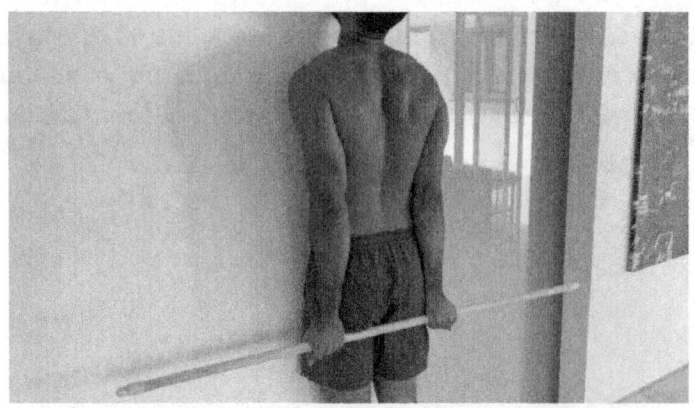

Start by standing with your feet hip-width apart, facing a wall. Hold a stick behind your back with both hands. Make sure your grip is firm, and your knuckles are facing away from the wall, with your palms facing towards your body. This grip is essential for maximizing shoulder extension. Engage your core and press your hips gently into the wall to keep your lower body stable.

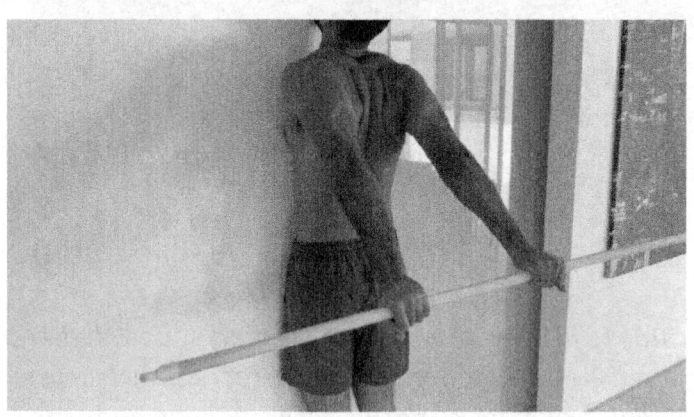

With your arms straight, slowly lift the stick as far back as possible, extending your shoulders and opening up your chest. Focus on moving your arms in a controlled manner while keeping your shoulders down and away from your ears. Once you've reached your maximum range of motion, hold the position for a moment to deepen the stretch, then slowly return to the starting position and repeat for reps.

The shoulder joint's remarkable range of motion is both a strength and a vulnerability. While it allows for incredible versatility in movement, it also requires careful attention to maintain its health and functionality. Neglecting shoulder mobility can lead to stiffness, imbalances, and an increased risk of injury, especially as we engage in more complex upper body exercises.

The exercises we've covered—such as stick shoulder dislocates and stick shoulder extensions—are essential tools for keeping your shoulders flexible, strong, and well-prepared for the demands of physical activity. By incorporating these mobilization exercises into your routine, you'll be taking important steps to protect your shoulder joints, improve your posture, and enhance your overall performance.

Remember, a well-rounded approach to upper body training is about ensuring that your joints are capable of moving freely and efficiently. Prioritizing shoulder mobility will help you avoid common injuries, achieve better results, and maintain a healthy, pain-free range of motion in your shoulders for years to come.

Programming Mobility For The Upper Body

The purpose of mobility training is to address the specific areas of your body that need work. I like combining these exercises into a routine that I use as a warm-up before my main workout. Depending on your level, you can do the same. Or, you can use this as a standalone workout on its own. We will dive in to the intricacies of how to program your workouts in Chapter 11, but for now you can experiment with how these different exercises feel for you so that you have awareness on what particular areas of your body need work.

Sample Upper Body Mobility Workout

Perform this workout as a standalone or as a warm-up for your main workout.

> 1. Wrist flexion: 1 set x 10 reps
> 2. Wrist extension: 1 set x 10 reps
> 3. Elbow rotation: 1 set x 10 reps
> 4. Elbow push ups: 1 set x 10 reps
> 5. Scapula push ups: 1 set x 10 reps
> 6. Rear scapula push ups: 1 set x 10 reps
> 7. Seated scapula lift: 1 set x 10 reps
> 8. Scapula pull ups: 1 set x 10 reps
> 9. Stick shoulder dislocates: 1 set x 8 reps
> 10. Stick shoulder extension: 1 set x 8 reps

Structural Balance For Sustainable Success

Throughout the last two chapters on creating alignment, we've emphasized one crucial idea:

Mobility is the foundation upon which strength is built.

Just as a building relies on a deep and stable foundation to rise high, your body depends on proper joint alignment and mobility to perform at its best.

In the last chapter, we began with the lower body, exploring the feet, ankles, knees, hips, and spine—the foundational elements that bear the greatest load and are often the first to compensate when alignment is lost. In this chapter, we turned our attention to the upper body, focusing on the scapula as the linchpin of upper body movement.

The overarching lesson is clear: without proper mobility, strength training can lead to compensations that strain the joints and increase the risk of injury. It's not enough to be strong;

you must also be aligned. Whether it's the knees compensating for tight hips or the shoulders struggling due to an immobile scapula, each joint's mobility directly impacts how your body moves as a whole. Through this journey, we've learned that alignment and mobility are the keys that unlock pain-free movement and the ability to sustain a lifelong fitness journey.

Charles Poliquin's Structural Balance Theory taught us that the body's strength lies in the balance between opposing muscle groups. As a coach, I've seen how neglecting the muscles of the back in favor of the mirror muscles creates imbalances that disrupt this structural balance, leading to common issues like shoulder impingement and chronic pain. The real problem often lies not in the muscles we can see but in those that are less visible—the stabilizers of the scapula, the muscles that control posture, and the joints that dictate alignment.

Developing scapular mobility is what ensures that your pushing and pulling movements are properly balanced, allowing you to engage your posterior chain effectively. The beauty of calisthenics is that it naturally requires total body engagement. When you have the awareness and control to engage the scapula, exercises like push ups and pull ups become opportunities to build balanced strength across the body.

In the next chapter, we'll dive into the specific strength training exercises that build upon a foundation of mobility. These exercises will not only increase your strength but also ensure that each rep is performed with optimal alignment, maximizing your results and protecting your joints.

Remember, strength built on poor mobility is a house of cards—it looks solid but collapses under pressure. True, lasting progress comes when your body moves as it was designed, with each joint supporting and balancing the others. As you move forward, continue to prioritize alignment and mobility. This approach will not only help you avoid the pitfalls of injury but also elevate your training, allowing you to reach new levels of strength and resilience.

Let's take the lessons from this chapter and apply them to the strength exercises that will carry you forward. The journey to a balanced, pain-free body begins with understanding how to move well. Turn the page, and let's dive into the strength side of the equation, ensuring every movement you make is grounded in the principles of alignment and mobility.

Chapter Takeaways

- When scapula mobility is compromised, the body compensates, often leading to pain in the shoulders, elbows, and wrists.

- Achieving balance between opposing muscle groups, particularly between the anterior (front) and posterior (back) chains, is critical for preventing injuries and optimizing performance.

- Developing scapular mobility ensures that the larger muscles of the back are doing their job, reducing the load on smaller muscles and joints like the biceps, elbows, and shoulders, which helps prevent common injuries.

- The beauty of calisthenics is that it inherently demands full-body engagement. By mastering scapular mobility, you unlock the potential for more efficient, aligned movement in every exercise.

CHAPTER 9 - THE SIMPLE SIX EXERCISES

"I fear not the man who has practiced 10,000 kicks once, but I fear the man who has practiced one kick 10,000 times."

—BRUCE LEE

He posted at 1:43 AM.

"Got 'The Men's Health Big Book Of Exercises,'" he wrote, the backlight of his screen throwing shadows across his ambition.

"733 exercises! Where do I even start?"

That final question echoed in the stillness of the late hour. It wasn't curiosity that laced his words, but a subtle plea—a search for direction in the overwhelm of 733 options.

Mastery is not a product of quantity but the repeated refinement of quality.

As a coach, I've witnessed the appeal of abundance cripple the potential for progress. Like a child at a beach trying to grab every pebble, we lose the chance to find the shells that truly matter.

With 733 exercises at his disposal, our community member stood at the brink of analysis paralysis, where the muscle of decision-making fatigues before a single rep is completed.

This is not just about the clutter of choice, but a misunderstanding of how our bodies are designed to move. Isolation is a fine detail tool, but the masterpiece of strength is painted with broader strokes—the simple six exercises. Push, pull, squat, hinge, rotation, and anti-rotation—these are the functional patterns that tell the story of human capability, where every muscle plays its part in a powerful symphony rather than a solo act.

The term "functional" has fallen victim to abuse over the years, losing the essence of its meaning in the fitness industry. Functional exercise is any exercise that works to achieve a chosen purpose or objective. Therefore, what is functional for a professional athlete may not be functional for a middle-aged weekend warrior because they are exercising for a different purpose and objective. What we will dissect in this chapter are the six key movement patterns that were necessary for survival in the developmental environment of our ancestors. In other words, without competency in these movements, it is unlikely you would survive in the wild. Our modern lifestyles are very different from those of our ancestors, but developing in these six movements is crucial for performing daily tasks with ease and staying injury-free.

I reached for my keyboard, the clack of the keys a call to simplicity.

"Focus on the patterns, not the parts," I began, my response cutting through the noise of 'more'.

"Your journey to strength isn't a page count. It's about mastering the movements that mirror life's demands. These are your compass in the wilderness of exercises."

In this chapter, we'll peel back the layers of complexity that have shrouded fitness in unnecessary confusion. You'll discover the liberating truth at the heart of effective exercise: less is indeed more. We'll dissect the six primal movement patterns and how these archetypal motions lay the foundation for a lifetime of strength, agility and mobility. You'll learn that by focusing on these six patterns, you can create a comprehensive training program that enhances every aspect of your physicality. For each pattern I will give you one exercise to build your body's capability through movements that translate into real-world functionality.

Through this lens, you'll see how a minimalist approach to exercise can lead to maximal gains. We'll discuss how to perfect these exercises, understand their variations, and how to program them effectively to achieve sustainable results.

By the end of this chapter, the fog of 'exercise overload' will clear, leaving you with a simple path forward. You'll be equipped with the knowledge to not just perform exercises, but to train with purpose and precision, paving the way for a stronger, more capable you.

Push: The Forward Force

Imagine our early ancestors, carving out a life in a world that demanded strength and resilience. Building shelters required the ability to push heavy objects, and clearing land for habitation involved pushing obstacles out of the way. In a fight, the strength to push an opponent could mean the difference between life and death. This primal movement pattern laid the groundwork for human survival and evolution.

Fast forward to today, and the relevance of pushing movements remains undeniable. Whether you're rearranging furniture, pushing a heavy door open, or shoveling snow from your driveway, the strength and stability developed through pushing exercises is indispensable. As we age, maintaining the ability to perform these movements becomes even more critical, ensuring we stay active, mobile, and independent over the long term.

PUSH UPS: THE MISUNDERSTOOD MASTERPIECE

The push up, an exercise we are all too familiar with, is frequently underestimated and misunderstood. When done right, it's a powerhouse that targets your chest, shoulders, and triceps, while engaging your core and offering isometric benefits to your back, spine, glutes, and quads. Executed correctly, push ups also cultivate stronger tendons, enhance joint health, and develop full-body coordination.

Steps to Perform a Proper push-up:

- Setup:
    1. Begin in a high plank position with your hands placed shoulder-width apart, slightly externally rotated. Slightly protract your scapula to create stability in your shoulder girdle.
    2. Maintain a posterior pelvic tilt to engage your glutes and core, preventing your lower back from arching.
    3. Fully extend your legs behind you with your feet together, engaging your quads to eliminate any knee bend, and keeping your body aligned from head to heels.

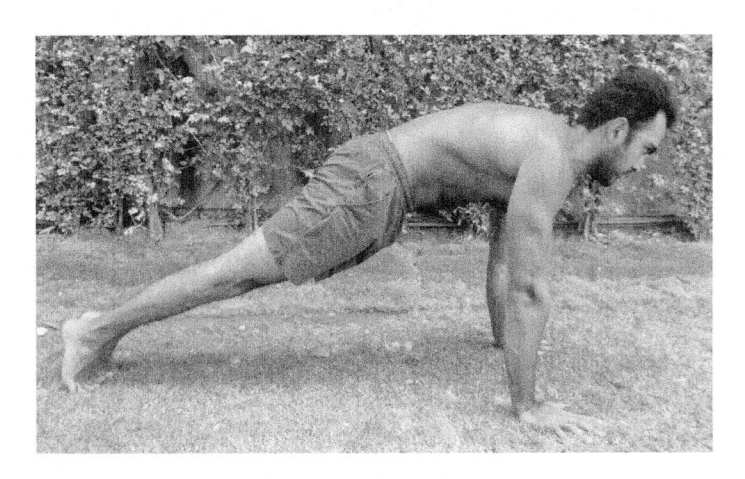

- Execution:
    1. Lower your body in a controlled motion by initiating scapular retraction. Keep your elbows at about a 45-degree angle to your body (not flared out or too close). Maintain alignment from head to heels by keeping your core, glutes, and quads engaged.
    2. As you reach the bottom, your chest should be just above the floor with elbows bent at approximately 90 degrees with the floor. Ensure your elbows aren't flaring out, and avoid letting your lower back arch.

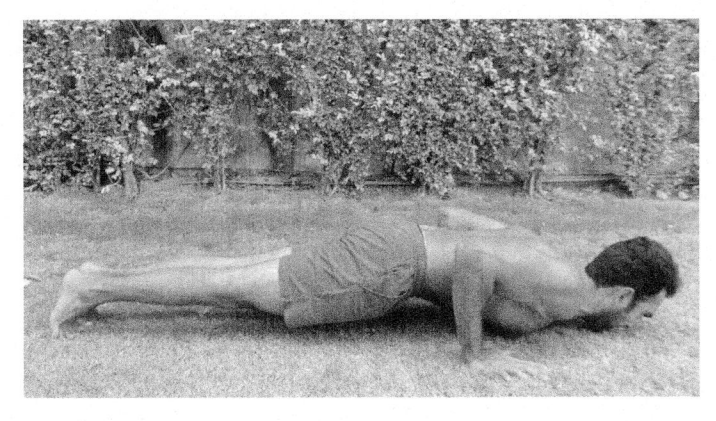

- Follow-through:
    1. Push through your palms and drive your

body back up to the starting position while maintaining the same alignment (glutes and core engaged, posterior pelvic tilt intact). Focus on engaging your chest, shoulders, and triceps as you press up.
2. Fully extend your arms at the top without locking your elbows, maintaining scapular protraction to keep your shoulders stable. Keep the tension in your core and glutes to reset for the next rep.

Early in my coaching career, I encountered a client we'll call Dana. Dana was in his mid-fifties and had spent years focusing on heavy weightlifting exercises like the bench press. Despite his impressive bench press numbers, Dana often complained of shoulder pain and wrist issues. He could lift heavy weights, but his joint mobility was lacking.

When I introduced Dana to scapula push ups (as discussed in the previous chapter) he struggled to perform even a few reps correctly. Despite having the pectoral, shoulder, and tricep strength for push ups, he lacked the neuromuscular ability to engage his scapula properly. This is something I've observed in many of my clients over my coaching career—developed muscular strength but lacking scapula mobility.

Dana's initial attempts at scapula push ups revealed his weaknesses, but with patience and consistent practice, he began to improve. Once he mastered the scapula push up, we moved to incline push ups. At first, Dana felt disheartened and expressed that he felt like a weak old man doing push ups at an incline. I reassured him, emphasizing that getting the form right and setting would provide the launching pad for his future gains.

Integrating the correct scapula movement into the incline push up took time, but when Dana finally got it, he understood the correct form for a full push up. His progress was significant; he could perform multiple sets with perfect form, and his wrist pain subsided. Dana reported feeling stronger and more capable in his everyday activities, such as pushing heavy doors open with ease, and noticed a significant improvement in his posture.

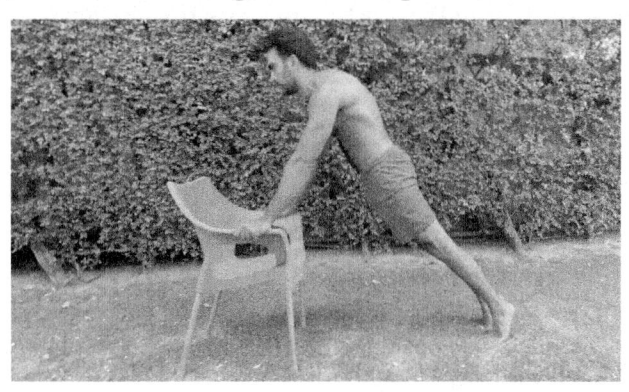

If regular push ups are too difficult for you right now, you can perform incline push ups by placing your hands on a chair (or other such sturdy object like a chest of drawers) that provides elevation to reduce intensity.

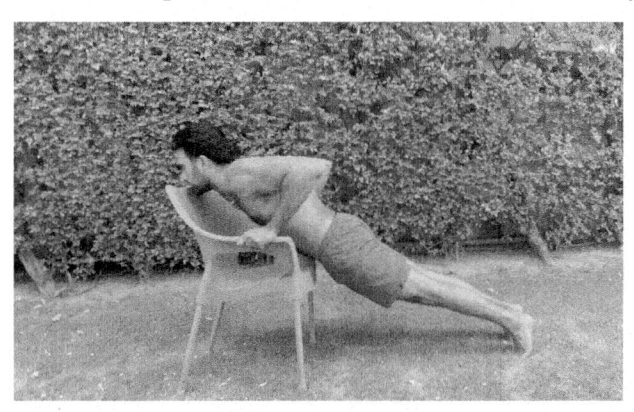

Go as low as you can at the bottom position, hold for a second, and then push back up to the starting position.

Remember, patience and precision are your allies. By dedicating time to perfecting your push up form, you lay the groundwork for all future strength and mobility gains. Embrace the journey of refinement, and your efforts will be rewarded with superior strength and functionality. Focus on building a body for life, not just for the next six weeks.

Pull: The Backward Brigade

In the journey of mastering the primal movement patterns, we transition from the assertive push to the equally vital pulling pattern. This movement is a connection to our primal roots and key to unlocking real-world strength.

Imagine the dawn of humanity. Our ancestors, much like the great apes, were masters of pulling, scaling trees with ease. This ancient movement, deeply ingrained in our DNA, is more than just an exercise; it's a reflection of our evolutionary heritage. When hunting for survival, our ancestors had to pull carcasses to safe places, often dragging them over long distances. Pulling heavy loads was a common task in their daily lives, and as humans developed watercraft, rowing became a vital movement, requiring significant pulling strength and endurance.

Today, the relevance of pulling movements remains critical. Whether you're carrying groceries, pulling a heavy door, or lifting your child into your arms, the strength and stability developed through pulling exercises are indispensable. Maintaining the ability to perform these movements is essential for staying active, mobile, and injury-free over the long term.

INVERTED ROW: GATEWAY TO PULL UP

The inverted row, often overlooked in favor of the more glamorous pull up, is a powerhouse for developing the upper back, shoulders, and biceps. It also engages the core and lower body, making it a full-body movement.

A unique aspect of the inverted row is its engagement of the spinal erectors. These muscles run along your spine and are crucial for maintaining an athletic posture. This exercise, essentially the opposite motion of the push up, serves as the gateway to proper execution of the pull up.

Steps to Perform a Proper Inverted Row:

- Setup:
    1. Lie flat on your back underneath a sturdy bar or table, legs extended, feet pointed, and heels on the ground. Grasp the bar or edge of the table with an overhand grip (palms facing away from you), hands about shoulder-width apart.
    2. Engage your core, glutes, and quads to keep your body aligned from head to heels. Let your shoulder blades fall into passive protraction (allowing them to spread apart slightly).

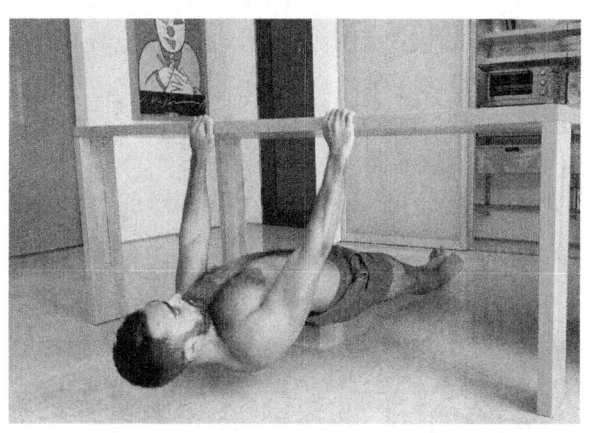

- Execution:
    1. Begin by retracting your scapula (pull your shoulder blades together) and initiate the row by pulling your chest towards the bar or table edge. Keep your elbows tucked at around a 45-degree angle from your torso.
    2. Pull until your chest is touching the bar or table. At the top, squeeze your shoulder blades together to fully engage your back muscles.

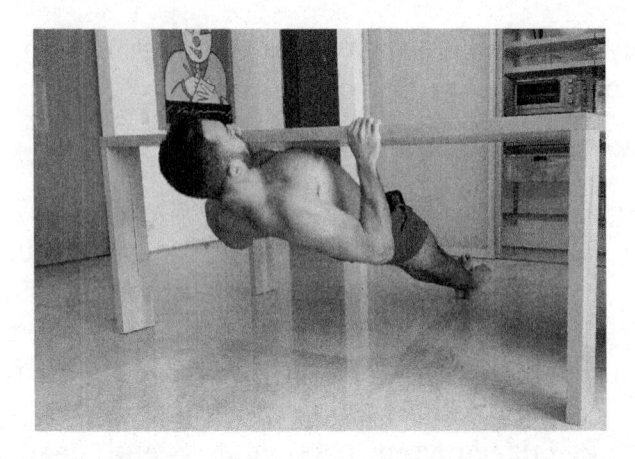

- Follow-through:
    1. Lower yourself back to the starting position in a controlled manner, keeping tension in your back and maintaining the straight line through your body. Allow your scapula to protract (spread apart) as you reach the bottom.
    2. Reset and repeat while ensuring your core and glutes remain engaged throughout the movement, keeping your body rigid.

Michael, my client I introduced you to in the last chapter, was determined to unlock pull ups because he saw them as the ultimate test of upper body strength. Before working with me, he had been attempting to do them on his own but stopped because of excruciating elbow pain. When I observed his exercise execution, I immediately noticed the issue. He had not learned how to properly engage his shoulder blades during the pull up which led his elbows to compensate and take on more load than they could handle.

I introduced Michael to the inverted row, explaining its importance as a foundational exercise for proper scapula engagement. Initially, he was overly reliant on his arms to complete the movement so we decreased intensity by having him bend his legs and use an underhand grip. As he learned to incorporate his shoulder blades, he noticed muscles working that he had never felt before. As a result, his posture improved, his upper back and rear delts became stronger, and the elbow pain he had experienced with pull ups started to diminish.

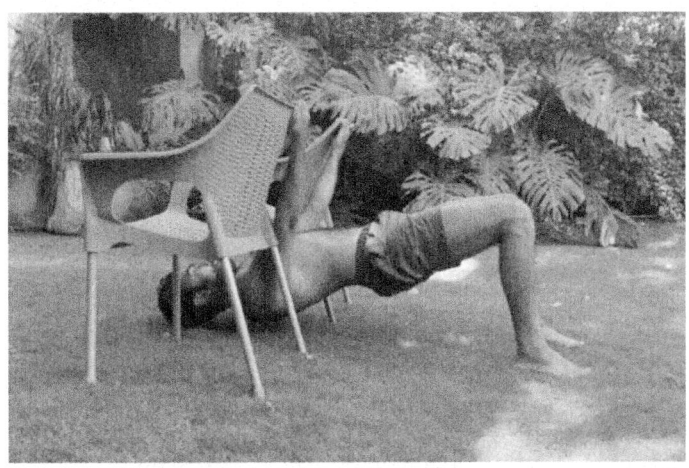

To decrease intensity on the inverted row, you can perform them with an underhand grip and legs bent.

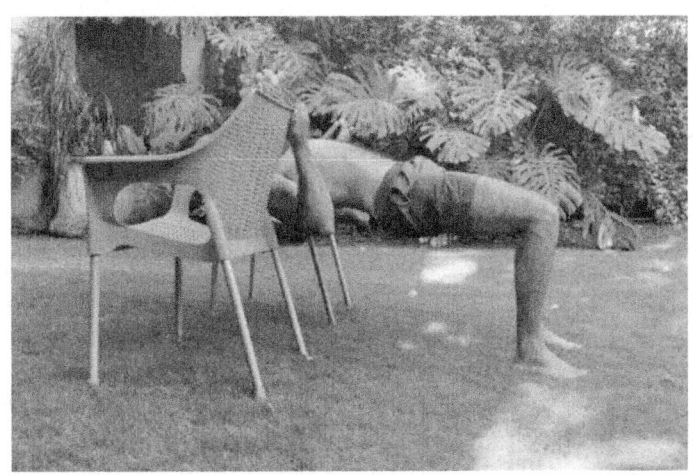

Initiate the motion with scapula retraction and pull all the way up to the point where your chest reaches wrist height before descending back to the starting position.

Over time, Michael mastered the inverted row, performing multiple sets with perfect form and even elevating his feet to increase intensity. When he was ready to start practicing pull ups, his form was significantly better, and he could perform them without pain. Michael's transformation highlights the necessity of mastering the inverted row before progressing to more advanced exercises.

The pull up is beyond the scope of this book because it is not a beginner exercise. Mastery of the basic inverted row forms the foundation for all pulling movements. Do not rush this process because poor form will lead to injury.

Squat: The Driving Force

When we think of strength, our minds often conjure images of broad shoulders and muscular arms. However, the true source of an athlete's strength lies in the lower body, specifically in the glutes, quads and hamstrings. This foundation is frequently overlooked, but without it, upper body strength cannot fully express itself.

For our early ancestors, squatting was an essential movement for survival. They had to squat to move heavy objects, build shelter, and even eat. Squatting was the original human sitting position, allowing for rest and stability in the absence of modern furniture. Today, however, many of us have lost this primal range of motion due to our sedentary lifestyles. Sitting on chairs and toilets that do not require our hips to go below our knees has contributed to a loss of flexibility and strength in the lower body.

Today, the squat remains critical for maintaining mobility and strength. Whether you're lifting heavy objects, climbing stairs, or getting up from a chair, the strength and stability developed through squatting exercises are indispensable.

ATG SPLIT SQUAT: ULTIMATE LOWER BODY EXERCISE

Squatting movements come in various forms, each targeting

different aspects of lower body strength and mobility. In this chapter, we will focus on one particular type of squat: the ATG (ass-to-grass) split squat. This variation emphasizes deep hip and knee flexion.

The ATG split squat is excellent for developing functional lower body strength that translates into everyday activities and athletic performance. It also improves balance, coordination, and hip mobility. This exercise also helps prevent common issues like lower back pain by lengthening the hip flexors.

We used to think that taking the knees over the toes was a bad thing. However, multiple studies have found that building the ability to fully bend the knee over time creates a more stable knee joint, thicker knee tendons, increased range of motion, and ultimately less chance of knee pain and injury. The majority of people have imbalanced legs and knees, where one leg may be more or less developed than the other. When we squat on two legs, these imbalances cannot be addressed effectively. The wonderful thing about the ATG split squat is that it trains one leg at a time, allowing for balanced development.

Additionally, the ATG split squat provides significant benefits to tight hip flexors, which often become shortened and weak due to modern lifestyles that involve excessive sitting. Normal squats may not effectively address this issue, but ATG split squats will. By lengthening the hip flexors and strengthening the surrounding muscles, this exercise helps restore proper hip function and alleviates discomfort associated with prolonged sitting.

Steps to Perform an ATG Split Squat:

Setup:
1. Begin in a staggered stance with one foot forward and the other foot back. Your feet should be about hip-width apart to maintain balance. Adjust the distance between your front and back foot to ensure you feel

comfortable and stable.
2. Keep your torso upright, with your back toes touching the floor and your heel elevated. Your chest should be open and facing forward.
3. Square your hips so they're facing directly forward, ensuring both are aligned evenly.

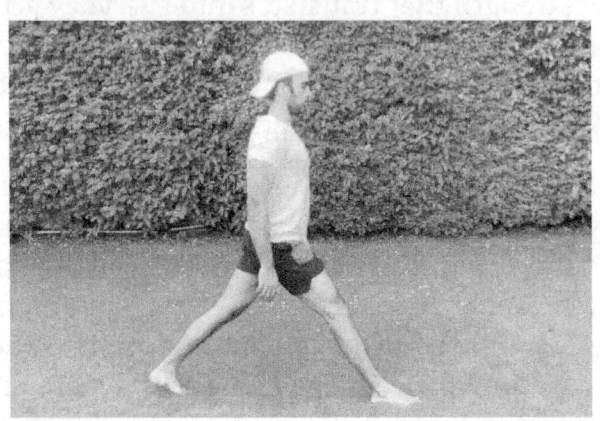

Execution:
1. Begin lowering your body by bending your front knee and maintaining an upright torso. Keep your back leg straight as you descend.
2. Allow your front knee to travel forward beyond your toes, focusing on maintaining control and alignment.
3. Continue lowering until your front hamstring fully covers your calf at the bottom position. Hold this position for a full second to ensure proper depth and engagement.

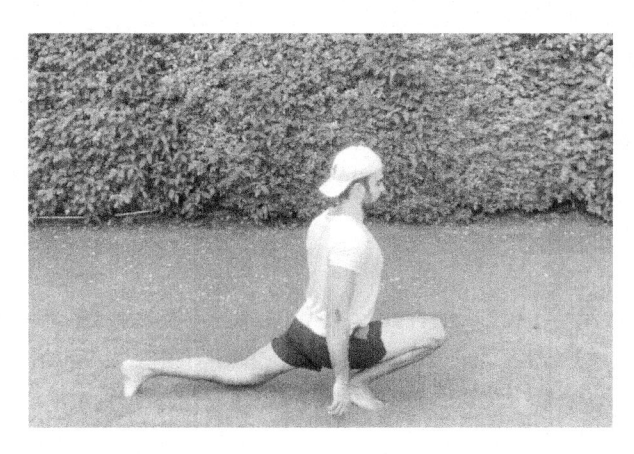

Follow-through:
1. Press through your front foot and drive back up to the starting position while maintaining control and alignment. Your torso should remain upright, and your hips square as you rise.
2. Reset your stance at the top and ensure both your core and legs are engaged before starting the next rep. Maintain your balance and focus on slow, controlled movement for each repetition.

For years, I struggled with chronic knee issues. I had torn cartilage in both knees, which severely limited my ability to engage in activities I loved, particularly combat sports. It was heartbreaking to be in the prime of my youth yet unable to train consistently because my knees would constantly cause issues and get tweaked. I wanted to immerse myself in martial arts, but felt weak and inadequate, unable to perform physically as a young man should.

I tried numerous approaches to heal my knees: physiotherapy, chiropractors, stretching, yoga—you name it, I tried it. Yet, nothing seemed to work. The isolated approaches I encountered failed to consider my body as an integrated unit. Faced with the prospect of surgery, where doctors would cut out pieces of my cartilage, I knew I had to find another way.

The guide who changed my path was Ben Patrick, who

introduced me to the ATG split squat. Through his programs and philosophies, I experienced a profound epiphany: the body functions as a single, integrated unit. My knee injuries were a result of compensations for tight hips. This realization opened a new opportunity to create strength through length, perfectly exemplified by the ATG split squat.

The ATG split squat contracts the quads, hamstrings, and glutes while lengthening the hip flexors, creating the supple strength we seek. This exercise challenges the conventional belief that taking the knees over the toes is harmful. In fact, mastering the ATG split squat means that those who can take their knees the furthest beyond their toes with control are the most protected against injury.

By mastering the ATG split squat, I transformed my legs into lean, athletic, and pain-free pillars of strength. Today, my knees are among my strongest joints, allowing me to train in combat sports consistently. This exercise taught me that we can rebuild weak areas, but it's crucial to understand the holistic process of how to do so.

Hinge: The Power Source

The hinge involves bending at the hips while keeping the back neutral. This fundamental movement pattern is crucial for developing strength and power in the posterior chain, which includes the glutes, hamstrings, and lower back.

Our early ancestors had to bend at the hips to gather food, lift heavy objects, and perform tasks necessary for building and maintaining their shelters. Hinging was vital for activities like digging and foraging, where the ability to move efficiently and powerfully from the hips was crucial.

In modern life, hinging remains important. Whether you're picking up a heavy box, lifting a child, or even just bending down to tie your shoes, the strength and stability developed through hinging is indispensable. Proper hinging technique also helps prevent common issues like lower back pain while making daily tasks easier and safer.

LYING HIP THRUST: BUILDING THE POSTERIOR CHAIN

We'll focus on the lying hip thrust as our primary exercise for developing the hinging movement pattern. This exercise strengthens the back side of the body while mobilizing the front side, promoting balanced strength and stability.

A unique aspect of the lying hip thrust is its ability to activate the glutes effectively, which is often neglected in modern lifestyles. Regular practice of this exercise helps develop awareness of how to engage your glutes, preventing compensations and enhancing overall functional strength.

Steps to Perform a Lying Hip Thrust:

- Setup:
    1. Lie flat on your back with your knees bent and feet hip-width apart, flat on the floor. Place your arms at your sides with your palms facing down for stability.
    2. Engage your core to maintain a neutral spine throughout the movement, ensuring your lower back doesn't arch as you begin.

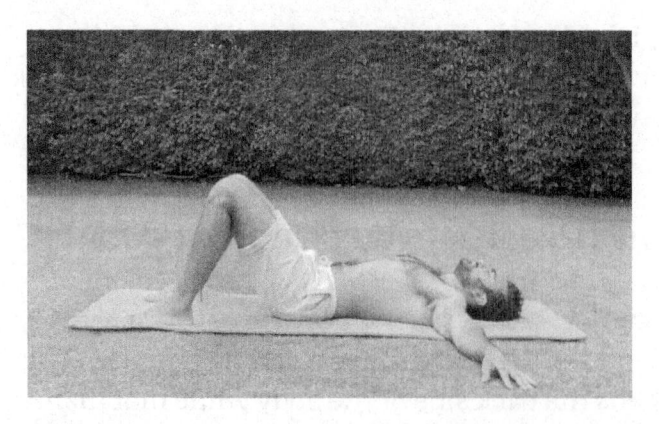

- Execution:
    1. Press firmly through your heels and lift your hips upward by contracting your glutes. Focus on driving the movement from your hips, not your lower back, to avoid strain.
    2. At the top of the movement, your body should form a straight line from your shoulders to your knees. Hold this position briefly, making sure to squeeze your glutes as tightly as possible.

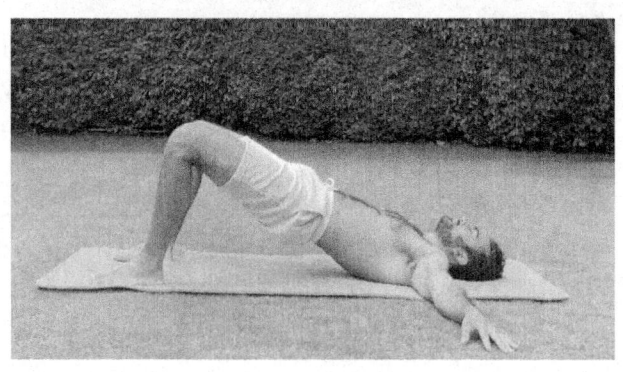

- Follow-through:
    1. Slowly lower your hips back to the starting position, maintaining control and keeping tension in your glutes and hamstrings. Avoid letting your hips drop too quickly or losing core engagement.
    2. Reset in the starting position with your glutes

still engaged and repeat the movement for the desired number of repetitions, focusing on form and control throughout.

Throughout my coaching career, I've encountered many clients who struggled with lower back pain due to poor hinging mechanics. One particular client, Alex, was a busy office worker who spent long hours sitting at a desk. He often complained of back pain and felt weak when performing simple tasks like lifting groceries.

I introduced Alex to the lying hip thrust, emphasizing the importance of engaging the glutes and maintaining a neutral spine. Initially, Alex found it challenging to activate his glutes properly. However, with consistent practice and focused attention on technique, he gradually improved.

Over time, Alex's hip thrusts became more powerful, and he noticed a significant reduction in his back pain. He reported feeling stronger and more confident in his daily activities. The lying hip thrust not only alleviated his discomfort but also allowed him to move more efficiently and safely.

By dedicating time to perfecting your hip thrust form, you ensure balanced posterior chain strength and improve your overall functionality. Focus on gradual progress and proper form to avoid setbacks and achieve sustainable results.

Rotation: The Core Catalyst

Rotation involves twisting the torso around the spine. This fundamental movement is crucial for developing core strength, stability, and flexibility, enhancing the efficiency of all other movement patterns.

For our early ancestors, rotational movement was vital for survival. Throwing a spear or swinging a club required efficient twisting, whether for hunting game or defending against threats. This ability to rotate the torso powerfully and efficiently was crucial for both offense and defense in a primal environment.

Today, the ability to rotate remains relevant for many daily tasks. Whether you're swinging a golf club, shoveling snow, or simply turning to grab something off the counter, rotational strength and flexibility are key.

This movement pattern helps stabilize the spine and transfer force from the lower body to the upper body, making it essential for both athletic performance and everyday activities. Rotational strength helps prevent back injuries, which are often the result of movements that combine twisting and bending.

The modern sedentary lifestyle often leads to tightness and immobility in the core and spine, increasing the risk of injury during activities that involve twisting. Addressing this tightness and improving rotational mobility is crucial for maintaining a healthy, functional body.

LYING LEG TWIST: ENHANCING ROTATIONAL ABILITY

We'll focus on the lying leg twist as our primary exercise for developing rotational strength and mobility. This exercise targets the core and spine, promoting balanced strength and mobility. Regular practice of this exercise helps develop awareness of how to engage the core and spine properly, preventing compensations and enhancing overall functional movement.

The lateral chain, which runs along the sides of your body, is a vital part of the body's movement system. While many people are familiar with the importance of the anterior chain (front) and posterior chain (back), the lateral chain is often overlooked. However, it's essential for twisting, rotating, and stabilizing the body during everyday movements and athletic activities.

The lying leg twist directly targets this area, focusing on the obliques, which power the rotational movement of the legs from side to side. In doing so, it enhances core strength, balance, and spinal mobility.

Rotation is a key function of the spine, allowing for twisting movements such as reaching, turning, or throwing. However, due to sedentary lifestyles and a lack of rotational training, many people experience stiffness in the spine, which can lead to compensatory movement patterns or even injury. The lying leg twist helps combat this stiffness by promoting a gentle, controlled rotation of the spine, improving its overall range of motion.

Additionally, this exercise mobilizes the hips by encouraging rotational movement in the pelvic region, further enhancing hip flexibility and coordination. The rotational motion also activates the muscles of the lower back and glutes, helping to keep the hips aligned while maintaining stability during the twist.

By regularly incorporating the lying leg twist into your routine, you improve the spine's rotational capacity, strengthen the lateral core muscles, and support overall spinal health. This increased mobility and strength not only enhances athletic performance but also helps prevent injuries by ensuring that the body can move freely and efficiently in all directions.

Steps to Perform a Lying Leg Twist:

- Setup:
    1. Lie flat on your back with your arms extended out to your sides, forming a 'T' shape with your body.
    2. Bend your knees and lift your legs so that your thighs are perpendicular to the ground and your lower legs form a 90-degree angle with your thighs (knees bent at 90 degrees).
    3. Engage your core, particularly your obliques, and

keep your lower back in a neutral position, pressed gently into the floor to prevent arching of the lower back as you perform the twist.

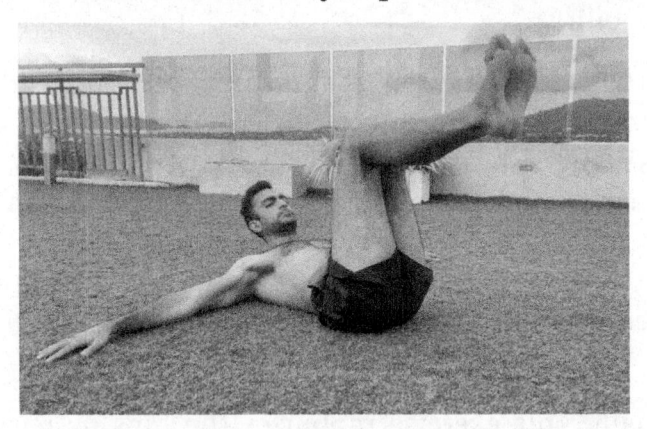

- Execution:
    1. Slowly lower your legs to one side, rotating your hips and allowing your knees to approach the ground on that side.
    2. As you lower, keep your shoulders pressed firmly into the floor to avoid excessive upper body rotation. Focus on controlled movement, using your obliques and core to lower the legs and maintain stability through the torso.
    3. Lower your legs towards the floor as you work to keep your shoulder on the opposite side connected to the floor. If you notice your shoulder rising, then don't go any lower.

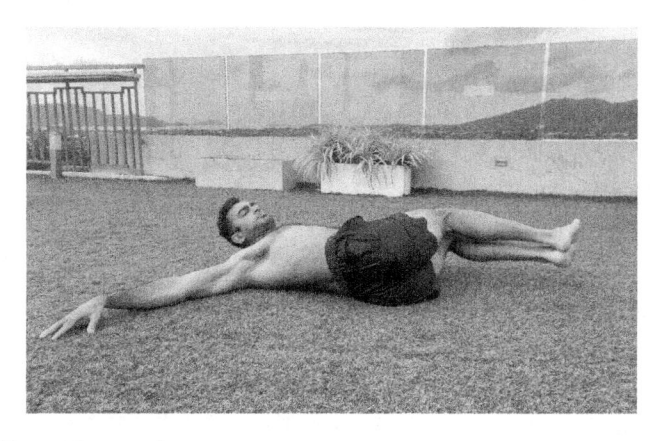

- Followthrough:
    1. Pause briefly at the bottom, feeling the stretch in your obliques and lower back, then engage your core and use your obliques to bring your legs back to the starting position.
    2. Repeat the movement on the opposite side, lowering your legs in the same controlled manner, focusing on spinal alignment and core engagement.

One of my clients, Tracy, was an avid golfer who struggled with back pain and limited range of motion. He loved the game but found it increasingly difficult to perform his best due to his physical limitations.

I introduced Tracy to the lying leg twist, emphasizing the importance of rotational mobility and core strength. Initially, he found it challenging to keep his shoulders flat on the ground and control the movement. However, with consistent practice and focused attention on technique, he gradually improved.

Over time, Tracy's rotational strength and flexibility increased significantly. He noticed a reduction in his back pain and an improvement in his golf swing. His increased range of motion allowed him to generate more power and control in his swings, enhancing his performance on the course.

Tracy's transformation highlighted the necessity of mastering the lying leg twist to improve rotational strength and mobility. This exercise not only alleviated his discomfort but also enhanced his overall functional movement, allowing him to enjoy his favorite activity pain-free.

Anti-Rotation: The Stabilizing Force

Where rotation is about producing rotational forces and enhancing core mobility, anti-rotation is about resisting those forces and maintaining core stability.

For our early ancestors, this ability was vital for tasks requiring a stable and strong core. Carrying heavy objects, climbing, and even defending against threats required the ability to maintain a stable torso, preventing unwanted twisting and potential injury.

In modern life, anti-rotation can help with carrying a heavy suitcase, pushing a shopping cart, or engaging in sports that require sudden changes in direction. Proper anti-rotation technique helps prevent injuries, especially in the lower back, by ensuring the core can resist unwanted movements and maintain stability.

HOLLOW BODY HOLD: BUILDING CORE STABILITY

The hollow body hold is a fundamental gymnastics exercise and is excellent for core stability. Lying on your backside body, flatten your lower back against the floor, maintain a rigid torso, and lift your legs up off the floor while raising your arms overhead. This position is a litmus test for core stability that protects your spine.

We'll focus on the hollow body hold as our primary exercise for developing anti-rotation strength.

Steps to Perform a Hollow Body Hold:

- Setup:
    1. Lie flat on your back with your arms extended overhead and your legs straight along the floor.
    2. Engage your core and press your lower back firmly into the ground. This helps eliminate any arching of your spine, which is key to the hollow body position.

- Execution:
    1. Lift your shoulders and arms off the floor while simultaneously raising your legs a few inches off the ground. Your body should form a slight curve, creating a "hollow" shape, with your lower back staying pressed against the floor.
    2. Keep your core muscles fully engaged, actively pressing your lower back down as you hold your arms and legs off the ground. The closer your arms and legs are to the floor without touching it, the more challenging the exercise becomes.

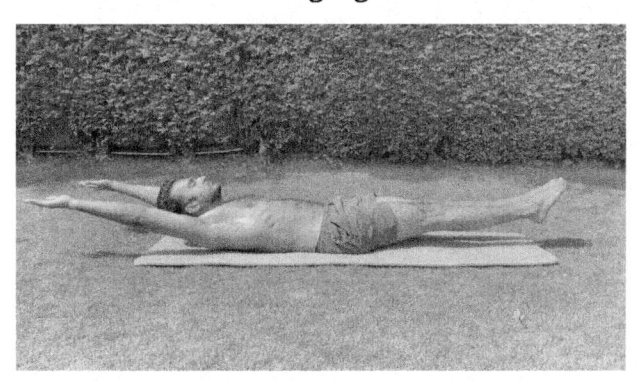

- Follow-through:
    1. Maintain this hollow position for the designated duration, focusing on keeping your core stable and avoiding any movement or shaking. Your arms and legs should remain extended, and your

lower back must stay glued to the floor.
2. Once you've reached the end of the hold, lower your arms, legs, and shoulders back to the ground in a controlled manner, keeping tension in your core until the very end. Reset before beginning another repetition if needed.

Locomotion: Movement Through Space

Locomotion is the ultimate expression of movement, encompassing the ability to move through space efficiently and effectively. It includes the basic forms of walking, jogging, and sprinting, collectively known as gait, as well as more complex movements like animal motions and acrobatics. Essentially, locomotion is the practical application of all the movement patterns we've discussed so far—push, pull, squat, hinge, rotation, and anti-rotation.

Our early ancestors had to move efficiently through various terrains to hunt, gather, escape threats, and migrate. All of this required a well-coordinated gait and the ability to traverse distances effectively. This necessity shaped the development of human movement and physical capabilities. In modern life, whether you're walking to the store, jogging to catch the bus, or sprinting in a game, the ability to move effectively and efficiently is crucial.

Locomotion also includes the playful and dynamic movements seen in animal exercises and acrobatics. These movements challenge our bodies in new ways, promoting creativity and adaptability in our physical capabilities.

The goal of mastering the simple six exercises—push up, inverted row, split squat, hip thrust, lying leg twist, and hollow body hold—is to enhance our ability to move through space efficiently. Locomotion, in essence, transcends and includes all these patterns, representing the pinnacle of physical capability and functional movement.

Programming The 'Simple 6'

There are many different ways to program the simple 6 exercises. As mentioned previously, you will get a complete guide to workout programming in Chapter 11. Until then, you can experiment with the sample workout provided below. I like the idea of training these exercises one after the other in a circuit because you can work to develop strength and stamina at the same time.

Sample 'Simple 6' Workout

Perform the following exercises in a circuit, i.e. one after the other with minimal rest between exercises and 3-5 minutes of rest between rounds.

1. Push up: 3 sets x 10 reps
2. Inverted row: 3 sets x 10 reps
3. ATG split squat: 3 sets x 10 reps
4. Lying hip thrust: 3 sets x 15 reps
5. Lying leg twist: 3 sets x 10 reps
6. Hollow body hold: 3 sets x 40-60 second hold

Mastering Movement

In this chapter, we embarked on a journey through the landscape of fundamental movement patterns that form the bedrock of effective calisthenics. We've identified the essential exercises and illustrated how each one plays a part in the larger framework for functional strength and athleticism.

Pushing teaches us the art of exerting force outward, building upper body strength and stability. Pulling balances our bodies and strengthens our grip on the physical world, enhancing our ability to draw objects towards us. Squatting provides the driving force, the foundation for every leap, bound, and sprint, by developing powerful legs. Hinging, as the power source, enables efficient bending and lifting, crucial for a strong posterior chain. Rotation enhances our core mobility, allowing us to twist and turn with ease, while anti-rotation focuses on core stability, resisting unwanted movements and protecting our spine. Finally, locomotion encompasses all these patterns, representing the mastery of movement through space.

Reflecting back to the opening story of our community member overwhelmed by the prospect of mastering hundreds of exercises, we now understand that true strength lies in simplicity and mastery. Bruce Lee's wisdom in fearing the man who has practiced one kick 10,000 times rather than 10,000 kicks once rings true in our approach to calisthenics.

By focusing on these fundamental movement patterns and exercises, we make every minute of our training count, cutting through the noise of endless exercise variety and focusing on what truly matters for strength, efficiency, and functional ability.

As we close the chapter on these simple six exercises, we transition to the 'Bodyweight Fitness Standards'. This upcoming guide is not just a roadmap but a compass that points you towards benchmarks of progression. In the next chapter, we will navigate with precision, understanding exactly where we are and what we need to do to elevate to the next level of physical development. We will define specific standards, measurable and attainable, for each stage of your growth.

It's time to go from understanding the 'what' and 'why' behind functional movements to understanding the 'how' of progression. Prepare to chart your course, to see the peaks of your potential, and to learn how to scale them one by one.

As you've learned the value of focus and mastery in your movements, you're now ready to apply those principles to a broader scale of development, marking your achievements and setting your sights on new heights. Welcome to the journey of physical evolution, where each step is clear, each milestone is defined, and the path to your next peak is laid out before you.

Chapter Takeaways

- Focusing on less exercises naturally creates faster progress because you're training your body to be most receptive to the same movement patterns again and again

- Exercises that stimulate multiple muscle groups and joints do the work of multiple isolation exercises at once, allowing you to move more weight and have a bigger impact on anabolic hormones.

- The simple six exercises – push up, inverted row, split squat, hip thrust, lying leg twist, hollow body hold – are the foundation for building strength and mobility.

- Building functional strength is about training in a way that makes you more effective in the real world, not just while exercising.

CHAPTER 10 - BODYWEIGHT FITNESS STANDARDS

"Your life is a reflection of your standards. If you set higher standards, you will elevate your life."

—TONY ROBBINS

Sam collapsed after doing a set of push ups to failure, his muscles burning with frustration. Three months of the same routine, and still, nothing. No progress in his form, no increase in reps, just the same old plateau. He stared at the ceiling, feeling stuck. As his eyes wandered, they landed on the glow of his gaming console in the corner. He remembered the rush of excitement when his character leveled up in his favorite RPG (role-playing game).

Why couldn't fitness feel like that?

That's when it hit him—*what if it could?*

Fitness doesn't have to be a grind. It can be a game—a real-life quest where each achievement unlocks new abilities, much like leveling up in a video game. By setting clear standards, your fitness journey becomes not just effective, but addictive.

In this chapter, I'm going to show you how to gamify your fitness and give you measurable standards to strive for. Just like in a game, each level has its own challenge—joint mobility, core stability, strength, cardio, and power—and you'll unlock new layers of fitness as you progress through them. Think of these as your quests, and each sign of progress releases a dopamine hit, keeping you hungry for more.

Each category of standards builds upon the one before it. While you can work on multiple areas simultaneously, always prioritize the foundational levels. For example, you can develop muscular strength while improving joint mobility, but never compromise joint health in the pursuit of strength because our joints are the foundation that support movement in general.

In this chapter, I will break down the fitness standards you need to focus on to level up in real life. We'll reference the Total Fitness Pyramid discussed in Chapter 5 and provide you with clear, measurable goals at each layer, starting from joint fluidity to explosiveness and power. Each standard builds on the previous one, ensuring you're progressing sustainably while avoiding injury.

Remember, lasting progress is a patient process. Rushing ahead can lead to setbacks through injury, as you may have experienced firsthand. Embrace the foundational standards as stepping stones—secure each one to confidently advance to the next.

Joint Fluidity Standards: Laying The Foundations

When building something meant to stand the test of time, the foundation is always the most important part. Without a solid base, everything that comes after is vulnerable to collapse. In fitness, that foundation is joint fluidity—the ability to move freely without pain or restriction. Whether you're in your 20s, striving to become an elite athlete, or in your 80s, focused on simply staying active, one thing will always matter most: how well your joints move.

For years, many—including myself—have been drawn to the allure of vanity in fitness: bigger biceps, ripped abs, heavier lifts. But those superficial markers quickly lose their value if your joints are constantly aching. What good is strength if it comes at the cost of daily discomfort? If you're experiencing pain in your wrists, elbows, shoulders, knees, or any other joint, focus on the specific exercises outlined in chapters 7 and 8 so you can prioritize reclaiming pain-free movement.

As for the basic joint fluidity standards, they are:

- Sitting-rising test: 10 points
- Scapula push ups: 10 reps
- Rear scapula push ups: 10 reps
- Seated scapula lifts: 10 reps
- Scapula pull ups: 10 reps

Scoring 10 points on the sitting-rising test (SRT) means lowering yourself to a seated position on the floor from standing and then standing back up again without relying on your arms, knees, or side legs for assistance. Points are deducted for each support used. The SRT reflects the mobility and flexibility of your ankles, knees, hips, glutes, hamstrings, calves, and back. Given that falls are a leading cause of death for those over the age of 65, it's no surprise that each point decrease on the SRT is linked to a 21% increase in death from all causes.

Executing upper body exercises like push ups, pull ups, dips, and rows with proper technique depends on your ability to properly engage your scapula. Without proper scapula engagement, compensations occur with aches, pains, and injuries being around the corner. This is why mastering the different positions of the scapula, as reflected in the standards above, is crucial.

Remember, longevity in fitness is not about the vanity of bigger muscles—it's about how well you can move, without pain, for the rest of your life.

Core Stability Standards: Establishing The Central Support

Just as a building relies on a strong central structure to prevent it from swaying or collapsing, your body depends on core stability to anchor every movement you make. Whether you're holding a plank, lifting a weight, or executing a jump, your core is constantly engaged, working behind the scenes to stabilize your body and prevent injury. Without this central support, even the strongest muscles in your body will lack control and coordination.

The following core stability standards provide the basic framework for strengthening your central support system:

- Anterior to posterior pelvic tilt: 10 reps
- Arch up hold: 60 seconds
- Hollow body hold: 60 seconds
- Side plank hold: 60 seconds
- Lying leg twist: 10 reps per side

The anterior to posterior pelvic tilt teaches you to control your pelvis positioning, which is essential for core engagement and spinal protection. The arch up hold stabilizes your posterior chain, the hollow body hold stabilizes your anterior chain, and the side plank hold stabilizes your lateral chains. The lying leg twist helps you build core stability through rotation.

Think of achieving these standards as establishing the central support that stabilizes a building. Without a stable core, your body's ability to perform and progress will be shaky at best. These standards are about ensuring that your body can move efficiently and powerfully, without compromising stability.

Strength Ability Standards: Building The Beams

With your foundation of joint mobility laid and your core stability in place as the central support, it's time to begin building the beams—the strength that will give your body the resilience and power it needs to handle the increasing demands of life and fitness.

These are the first set of strength ability standards to accomplish:

- Push ups: 15 reps
- Inverted rows: 12 reps
- ATG split squats: 10 reps per side
- Lying hip thrusts: 15 reps

When you can pump out 15 reps of push ups with perfect form, then you will be ready for more advanced pushing exercises like dips. Similarly, when you're able to achieve the inverted row standard from a body position that is nearly horizontal to the floor, then you will be ready for more advanced pulling exercises like pull ups. Mastering ATG split squats will prepare you to take on single-leg squats and lying hip thrusts will teach how to properly activate your glutes and hamstrings. Dips, pull ups, and single-leg squats are beyond the scope of this book, but mastering the above standards will serve as stepping stones for safely progressing towards them.

Working on these standards will add muscle mass to your chest, back, and limbs. The more muscle you add, the denser your bones will get in order to support it. So this is kind of like building the beams that will allow your body to stay strong through motion. The stronger your beams, the more confidently you can progress in your fitness journey, knowing your body is built to last.

Cardio Capacity Standards: Fortifying The Framework

Now that the beams of strength are in place, the next critical step in building a body that can stand the test of time is fortifying the framework with cardio capacity. Just as a building's framework must be reinforced to withstand external pressures and environmental challenges, your body needs cardiovascular endurance to sustain effort and maintain strength over time.

Cardio capacity is your body's ability to efficiently deliver oxygen to your muscles during sustained activity, allowing you to endure longer periods of physical exertion without fatigue. It's what gives you the stamina to keep going, whether you're tackling a long hike, a high-intensity workout, or simply moving through a busy day.

The most common and effective way to measure this endurance is through VO_2 max, which reflects the maximum amount of oxygen your body can utilize during exercise. The higher your VO_2 max, the better your cardiovascular system is at supporting prolonged physical activity. Improving this capacity ensures that your body can maintain its structure and strength, even under increasing demands.

How to approximate your VO_2 max at home

$$VO_2 \text{ max} = 15.3 \times (HR_{max}/HR_{min})$$

1. Approximate your maximum heart rate by subtracting your age from 220.
2. Determine your resting heart rate by placing two fingers on the pulse in your throat and count your beats per minute.
3. Divide your maximum heart rate by your resting

> heart rate.
> 4. Once you have the result of that division, multiply by 15.3.
> 5. Compare your current VO₂ max to the norms for men provided in the following table.
>
> For example:
>
> If $HR_{max}=165$ and $HR_{min}=80$
>
> VO_2 max = 15.3 x (165/80)
>
> VO_2 max = 31.55 ml/kg/min

Below is a table showing VO₂ max percentiles for men across different age groups. This table allows you to assess where you are now and set goals for improvement:

VO2 MAX PERCENTILES MEN

AGE GROUP	5TH PERCENTILE	10TH PERCENTILE	25TH PERCENTILE	50TH PERCENTILE	75TH PERCENTILE	90TH PERCENTILE	95TH PERCENTILE
20-29	29	32.1	40.1	48	55.2	61.8	66.3
30-39	27.2	30.2	35.9	42.4	49.2	56.5	59.8
40-49	24.2	26.8	31.9	37.8	45	52.1	55.6
50-59	20.9	22.8	27.1	32.6	39.7	45.6	50.7
60-69	17.4	19.8	23.7	28.2	34.5	40.3	43
70-79	16.3	17.1	20.4	24.4	30.4	36.6	39.7

As you can see, VO₂ max max naturally declines with age, but that doesn't mean you should settle for the average. Striving for a VO₂ max above 55 ensures that you're not just surviving but thriving. It's the key to longevity and performance, allowing you to continue progressing in your fitness journey without losing steam.

By working on your cardio capacity, you're fortifying your body's framework, ensuring it can handle more demanding workouts and sustain effort over long durations. Whether you prefer running, swimming, cycling, or high-intensity interval training (HIIT), all of these activities can help elevate your VO_2 max and improve your overall endurance.

With a strong cardiovascular system in place, your body is equipped to handle the dynamic demands of both strength and endurance.

Muscle Elasticity Standards: Generating Power

With the foundation, central support, beams, and framework all in place, the last phase in constructing a body built to stand the test of time is developing power. Power is the ability to generate force and elasticity in your muscles—allowing you to move explosively, with speed and strength. This is the final layer, the dynamic element that turns strength into action.

The standard for power is simple but challenging:

- All-out sprint for 30 seconds.

While this may sound straightforward, sprinting is one of the most powerful expressions of muscle elasticity, requiring full-body coordination and explosive force.

However, there's an alarming statistic: 90% of people never sprint again after the age of 30. Once we stop engaging in these fast-twitch, explosive movements, we begin to lose that elasticity in our muscles. And when elasticity fades, the aging process speeds up. Without that spring-like ability to generate quick bursts of energy, our bodies become stiffer, slower, and more prone to injury.

Sprinting is more than just a display of speed—it's a marker of youth and vitality. The ability to sprint taps into the fast-twitch muscle fibers, keeping them active and preventing the body from slipping into the decline that comes with age. By incorporating regular sprint work into your fitness routine, you're doing more than just increasing your power; you're maintaining the elasticity that will keep you moving dynamically as you age.

The key is to approach this standard with safety and progression in mind. Start by gradually increasing your sprint intervals and build up to that full 30-second, all-out effort. This ensures that your joints, muscles, and tendons are prepared to handle the intensity of sprinting without injury.

Incorporating sprints keeps your body adaptable and resilient, much like how a well-built structure can withstand the shocks and pressures of its environment. Sprinting not only trains your muscles but also reinforces everything you've built—mobility, stability, strength, and endurance—bringing it all together in one powerful movement.

The Power Of Standards

In life, having clear standards sets the foundation for progress. Whether in fitness, relationships, or career, standards give you measurable targets to work toward and serve as the guideposts that keep you on track. Without standards, it's easy to drift, to fall into complacency, and to never truly reach your potential.

In fitness, standards are essential because they define what you should aspire to in order to create a strong, resilient, and functional body. These standards aren't just about what you can achieve now—they are about laying the groundwork for sustained health, longevity, and well-being. By focusing on mobility, stability, strength, endurance, and power, you ensure that your body is built to not only handle today's challenges but also those of the future.

Standards provide you with a clear direction, helping you measure where you are now and where you need to go. They prevent stagnation by continually giving you something to work toward. Whether you are a beginner or advanced, the process of continually meeting and surpassing standards ensures that you are always progressing.

Just as in any area of life, holding yourself to standards in fitness brings purpose and clarity to your efforts. It ensures that every step you take is intentional and aligned with your long-term goals.

Now that you understand the importance of having clear standards, the next step is to create a routine that aligns with them. In the next chapter, we'll dissect the 8 variables of programming, giving you the tools to design a fitness plan that's tailored to your goals, your schedule, and your unique needs.

Chapter Takeaways

- Pain-free movement is the most important attribute of fitness. Prioritize mobility training to ensure your body can move freely without restriction.

- Core stability is your central support. A strong core anchors all movement, providing balance, coordination, and injury prevention.

- Strength provides the structure your body needs to handle physical demands with control and resilience.

- Improving your cardiovascular capacity ensures that your body can sustain prolonged physical activity.

- Sprinting and other explosive movements preserve the muscle elasticity that keeps your body dynamic and youthful, even as you age.

- Setting clear standards for each area of fitness gives you measurable goals, ensuring that you continue to improve over time.

- Focusing on mobility, stability, strength, endurance, and power creates a well-rounded approach to fitness that supports you for life.

CHAPTER 1
CONSTRUCTING YOUR ROUTINE

"You have your way. I have my way. As for the right way, the correct way, and the only way, it does not exist."

—FRIEDRICH NIETZSCHE

"I've hit a wall," the message began, a clear note of frustration echoing through each typed word.

A member of our community, someone who had been enthusiastically following a routine from a popular Instagram influencer, had posted in our forum. His journey, which started with promise and excitement, had taken an unexpected turn.

"I followed the routine to the letter," he continued, "but my shoulders can't take it anymore and I can barely do a push up without pain."

As I read his message, I felt the emotion in his words. He wasn't just hitting a physical barrier; he was confronting a realization that his efforts, though earnest, might have been misguided. His

...signaling a distress call, urging him to stop, hinting ...nething fundamental was missing. This is where we ... our exploration in this chapter.

...o two people are exactly the same. We all have different body types, physical abilities, goals, schedules and preferences. A successful training program accounts for these individual differences. Remember the *Law of Individuality* discussed earlier in Chapter 6? In this chapter we will put this law into practice. The internet is filled with cookie-cutter plans, but a personalized approach will always produce the best results.

In this chapter, you will discover the eight variables of personalized training. Adjusting these variables is how you will create a routine that resonates with and responds to your unique body type, situation and goals.

By the end of this chapter, you will have the tools to construct a routine that is as unique to you as your fingerprint, ensuring that your fitness journey is both effective and sustainable.

The Eight Variables Of Personalized Training

Searching for the perfect routine can feel like searching for a shadow in the dark—it's there, but you need the right light to see it. That light is cast by the eight training variables, each one a dial to tune your workout to the unique frequency of your body type and goals. These are your tools to carve out success from the stone of effort.

Variable #1 - Exercise Selection

Exercise selection is the process of choosing specific exercises to include in your workout program. This is the most important aspect of your training routine because it dictates the direction and effectiveness of your journey. Adjusting this variable means choosing the exercises that align with your personal fitness goals, current physical condition, and long-term aspirations.

The significance of exercise selection lies in the *Law of Specificity*, or SAID (specific adaptations to imposed demands). Remember from Chapter Six that your body adapts to the type of demands you place upon it. Therefore, the exercises you select directly influence the kind of results that follow.

If your primary focus is on building a foundation of mobility and core stability, then your exercise selection should reflect that goal. Alternatively, if your primary goal is muscle and strength gain, then the exercises must be aligned with that objective. This tailored approach ensures that every movement and every rep contributes meaningfully towards your specific fitness targets.

How to Select the Right Exercises

- Assess your current level: Do you have the hip mobility to enter into a full deep squat position? Do you have the core stability to hold the hollow body position for a minute? Can you perform 15 clean reps of full range of motion push ups without pain? Use the framework shared in the previous chapter on the bodyweight fitness standards as a reference.

- Consider your limitations: Do you have any physical limitations or areas of concern? For instance, if you have weak wrists, then include exercises in your routine to strengthen them. If your pulling strength is much weaker compared to your pushing strength, then prioritize pulling movements to build structural balance. This ensures that your routine not only helps with overall development but also addresses specific weak links to prevent injury.

- Align with your goals: Are you training to improve performance in a specific sport? Do you want to gain as much muscle as possible? Are you looking to alleviate painful joints? Each exercise you choose should be a stepping stone towards your desired outcome.

- Seek balance: Ensure your routine is well-rounded. This means incorporating exercises that target all the different muscle groups so that no body part is neglected. A balanced routine prevents overuse injuries and promotes full-body development.

- Stay open to adjustment: Be prepared to modify your exercise selection as you progress. As your body adapts and your capabilities evolve, so too should your routine. This adaptive approach keeps your training effective and engaging.

By selecting exercises tailored to your specific stage of development, goals, and physical needs, you lay the groundwork for a successful and sustainable fitness journey. The right selection of exercises is the first step in constructing your personalized routine.

Variable #2 - Exercise Order

Exercise order is the sequence in which you perform exercises during a workout. This aspect of your routine is about much more than organization; it's a strategic choice that impacts the effectiveness of your training and the specific adaptations your body will undergo.

The order in which you perform your chosen exercises will shape the specific physical improvements you'll see. By thoughtfully sequencing exercises, you can ensure that each one is performed when your energy and concentration are at their peak, leading to better technique, higher intensity, and more effective training.

For instance, if you have an imbalance where your upper body is more developed than your lower body, then prioritizing exercises can help address this. Exercising your lower body before your upper body, when you're less fatigued, allows for more focused effort on developing under trained muscles, promoting structural balance.

Similarly, if certain movements cause discomfort, like wrist pain during push ups, arranging your routine to include preparatory exercises as a form of prehab can help warm up and lubricate your joints before more strenuous activity.

How to Select the Right Order of Exercises

- Assess your strengths and weaknesses: Identify which areas need more focus. If you have a more developed chest compared to your shoulders, then start with pike push-ups instead of regular push ups to balance your development.

- Prioritize your goals: For instance, if you're looking to improve performance in tennis then prioritizing pushing exercises makes sense for your sport. On the other hand, if you're looking to improve performance in climbing then prioritizing pulling exercises makes more sense.

- Consider fatigue and intensity: Place demanding or high-intensity exercises at the beginning of your workout when you're less fatigued. This approach ensures proper technique and reduces risk of injury.

- Warm-up and prehab: Include exercises that prepare your body for the workout, especially if you have areas prone to discomfort or injury. For example, incorporating wrist mobility exercises before push-ups can help alleviate wrist pain.

- Adapt to feedback: Be attentive to how your body responds to the order of exercises. If you notice certain patterns, like consistent fatigue impacting your performance in a key area, don't hesitate to adjust the sequence accordingly.

- Balance and variety: Ensure that your routine is balanced, alternating between different muscle groups and types of movements to prevent overuse and maintain engagement.

Tailoring the sequence of exercises in your routine to your unique needs and goals transforms your workout from a generic set of movements into a personalized path to success.

Variable #3 - Number Of Sets

The number of sets in a workout is the collection of repetitions performed on a particular exercise separated by rest periods. It's a component in determining the total volume of your workout (volume = sets x reps x intensity).

The amount of sets you perform has a direct impact on muscle growth, strength development, and neurological adaptations. While research on the ideal number of sets for muscle growth and strength gains is not conclusive, the key takeaway is that individual response differs greatly.

For increasing muscle size, some studies suggest that multiple sets work well in providing enough stimulus for growth and adaptation. Other studies conclude that a single set of an exercise performed to failure is all that's required for muscle growth. When it comes to strength, however, we must also account for the impact of neurological adaptations.

Recall from Chapter Four that strength is expressed as a combination of muscle size and muscle fiber recruitment by the nervous system. Even if multiple sets don't directly contribute to muscle growth, they do train your nervous system to become more efficient at recruiting muscle fibers. In other words, neuromuscular adaptations enhance your efficiency in movement patterns and muscle recruitment so that you can express your strength more fully. Therefore, considering the number of sets is not just about muscle growth; it's about developing strength as a skill.

How to Select the Right Number of Sets

- Assess your current stage: Your level of fitness significantly influences the ideal number of sets. As a beginner, performing multiple sets works well to integrate the fundamental movement patterns into your nervous system and build connective tissue strength. At more advanced levels, performing fewer sets may work better for building strength.

- Align with your goals: Adjust the number of sets to your specific objectives. If your focus is on building muscle, you might lean towards higher sets. For strength and skill development, the emphasis should be on the quality of each set rather than quantity.

- Balance intensity and volume: Higher intensity workouts (requiring more effort per set) should have fewer sets to avoid excessive stress, while lower intensity workouts can have more sets.

- Consider overtraining risks: Be mindful of the point of diminishing returns. Multiple sets that exceed your body's capacity for recovery lead to overtraining. If you're hitting a plateau, sometimes the solution is not more sets but rather allowing more time for recovery.

- Experiment and adapt: Since the ideal number of sets varies greatly from person to person, experimentation is key. Try different set ranges and monitor how your body responds. Adjust accordingly based on your recovery, progress, and any signs of overtraining.

- Maintain overall balance: Ensure that the total number of sets per workout is manageable and sustainable. This balance helps in maintaining consistency and long-term progress without burnout.

Adjusting the number of sets per exercise in your workout ensures that every set contributes to your journey towards achieving your fitness goals, whether it's muscle growth, strength, or mastering specific skills.

Variable #4 - Intensity

Intensity can be viewed in two ways:

1) As the objective level of resistance used in an exercise, and
2) As the subjective perception of effort during the exercise, regardless of the actual resistance.

Objectively, doing 25 reps of standard push ups requires a certain amount of effort if two people weigh the same. But subjectively, doing 25 reps can be more or less intense depending on the strength of the person performing the exercise. For this reason, we will view intensity subjectively as the degree to which your muscles are challenged.

Generally speaking, higher intensity training is better for muscle and strength gains, while lower intensity training is better for improving stamina and endurance.

Understanding the right intensity is particularly important in calisthenics because unlike in weight training where we can easily increase or decrease the amount of weight lifted, our body weight remains more or less the same on any given day. Therefore, we must adjust intensity by making an exercise more or less challenging.

How to select the right intensity

- Use RM (repetition maximum): RM is a useful measure of intensity. If a training program tells you to perform an exercise for 8-15 RM, then you choose a variation that allows you to perform at least 8 but no more than 15 repetitions. For instance, if you are easily able to perform more than 15 standard push ups, then increase intensity by switching to a more challenging variation (like side-to-side push ups).

- Apply the OMNI-Resistance Scale: This subjective 10-point scale measures your rating of perceived exertion (RPE). Each number on the scale represents ~10% of your maximum effort. A rating of 10 means maximum effort (to failure), while a rating of 8 suggests stopping at 80% of your maximum capacity. For example, if 10 pull ups is the maximum number of repetitions you can perform and a routine tells you to go for an RPE of 8, then that means stopping at 8 reps to leave 2 reps in the tank so that you can accumulate more volume over multiple sets rather than going to failure.

- Adapt based on ability: Your current fitness level should guide your intensity choice. If you struggle with a basic version of an exercise, reduce the intensity to a more manageable level so that you can accumulate more reps and train your nervous system to learn the movement. Conversely, if an exercise feels too easy, increase the challenge to continue making muscle and strength gains.

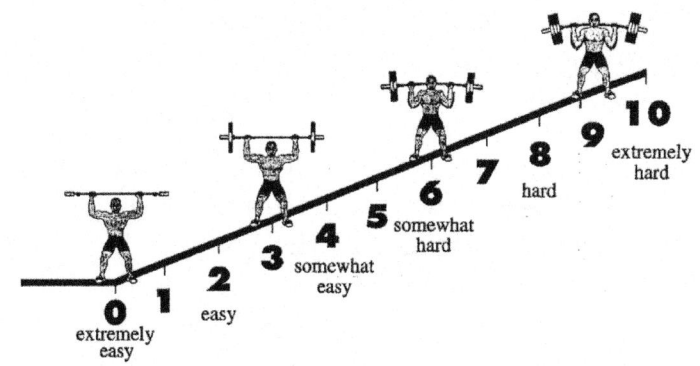

The OMNI resistance scale measures your subjective rating of perceived exertion (RPE) from 0 to 10 on a particular exercise.

- Balance intensity with other variables: Intensity should be balanced with the number of sets and reps you're doing.

Higher intensity generally means fewer reps and sets, while lower intensity can accommodate more volume.

- Monitor your body's response: Pay attention to how your body responds to different levels of intensity. If you're constantly fatigued or not making progress, adjust the intensity accordingly. Remember, it's about finding what works best for you, not blindly following predetermined standards.

- Be flexible and patient: Intensity isn't static; it can and should change as you progress in your fitness journey. Be open to adjusting as your body grows stronger and more capable.

Selecting the right intensity for your exercises is a blend of understanding your capabilities and challenging yourself appropriately. It's a dynamic process that requires tuning in to your body's signals and adapting as you progress, ensuring each workout is effectively contributing to your fitness goals.

Variable #5 - Repetitions

Repetitions, or 'reps,' refer to the number of times you perform an exercise in a set. The number of reps is inversely linked to intensity, i.e. higher intensity means that a fewer number reps can be performed.

Understanding reps is key to tailoring your workout to your goals because different rep ranges impact various aspects of physical fitness. The concept of the conditioning continuum helps provide further clarity:

CONDITIONING CONTINUUM

```
      1-5 REPS      6-15 REPS      >15 REPS

     STRENGTH      HYPERTROPHY     STAMINA
```

- 1-5 RM range: When the intensity is high enough to keep you from going beyond 5 reps, then the emphasis is on neuromuscular components of strength. Keeping reps between 1-5 is best for developing explosive strength and power.

- 6-20 RM range: When the intensity is low enough to allow for at least 6 reps and high enough to stop you from going beyond 20 reps, then the focus is on hypertrophy (aka muscle growth). Keeping reps between 6-20 reps is beneficial when prioritizing muscle growth.

- Beyond 20 Reps: When the intensity is low enough to allow for more than 20 reps on a particular exercise, then you are primarily training stamina to enhance muscular endurance and cardiovascular fitness.

Keep in mind that the conditioning continuum is not a rigid rule. Training in the 1-5 rep range, while emphasizing power generation, can also contribute to hypertrophy. Working beyond 20 reps, while primarily building stamina, can also impact muscle growth.

How to Select the Right Number of Reps

- Understand muscle fiber types: Different muscle fibers respond differently to rep ranges. Type I fibers (aka slow twitch fibers) are suited for stamina and are trained through higher reps at lower-intensity. Type II fibers (aka fast twitch fibers) have high force production but quick fatigue rate and are trained through high-intensity, low-rep workouts.

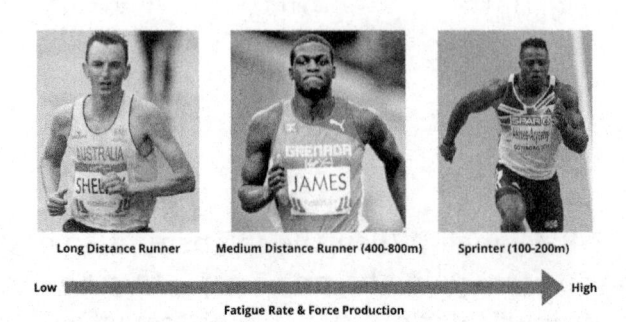

| Long Distance Runner | Medium Distance Runner (400-800m) | Sprinter (100-200m) |

Low ──────────────────────────────► High
Fatigue Rate & Force Production

Long distance runners train to develop Type I fibers that have ~100 muscle fibers per unit. Sprinters train to develop Type II fibers that have ~10,000 muscle fibers per unit. This difference between the amount of muscle fibers per unit is why sprinters are more muscular than long distance runners.

- Align reps with goals: Choose your rep range based on your objectives. If your primary goal is to build explosive power, train with lower rep ranges (1-5 RM). For muscle growth, aim for the 6-20 RM range.

- Consider orderly recruitment: This principle states that lower intensity exercise primarily trains slow-twitch muscle fibers, while higher intensity exercise primarily trains fast-twitch muscle fibers. Select reps and intensity that align with the muscle fibers you aim to develop.

- Balance rep ranges for full-body fitness: To develop complete fitness, incorporate a variety of rep ranges into your routine to ensure that you're building strength, hypertrophy, and stamina effectively.

- Adjust based on current fitness level: Your current level of fitness will dictate the most effective rep range for you. A beginner will benefit from higher reps at lower intensity to build endurance and technique, while an advanced trainee might focus on lower reps at higher intensity for strength gains.

- Be flexible and adaptive: As your body adapts and your fitness level changes, be ready to modify your rep ranges. Continuously assess and adjust your training to ensure ongoing progress and prevent plateaus.

By adjusting the number of repetitions for each exercise, you create a workout that is precisely calibrated to your goals and current level. This approach ensures that every rep you perform is a step towards achieving your desired physical transformation.

Variable #6 - Rest Period Between Sets

Rest periods between sets is the amount of time you take to recover after completing one set and before starting the next set. This variable is important because it directly influences your performance in each set and the overall effectiveness of your training session.

Rest periods play a role in determining the energy systems your body utilizes during a workout and how it recovers. For high-intensity, low-rep sets, longer rest periods are necessary to replenish the anaerobic energy systems, primarily the ATP-PC system, which is responsible for short bursts of high energy.

Conversely, shorter rest periods, particularly in circuit-style training, enhance stamina. They keep your heart rate elevated and challenge your body's ability to recover quickly, providing a different kind of stimulus compared to strength or power training.

How to Select the Right Amount of Rest Between Sets

- Match rest periods to intensity: As a general rule, the

higher the intensity (i.e. lower reps), the longer your rest period should be between sets. This allows for adequate recovery of your energy systems and ensures you can maintain high performance in each set.

- Tailor to training goals: If your goal is to maximize power generation, opt for longer rest periods (up to five minutes) between sets to allow for full recovery of the ATP-PC system. If your goal is to improve stamina or cardiovascular fitness, shorter rest periods (10 seconds to two minutes) are more appropriate.

- Consider your fitness level: As you progress from the Novice to Warrior level (as discussed in the previous chapter) you might shift from individual sets with rest to a circuit-style workout with minimal rest. Adjust your rest periods based on your current fitness level and training phase.

- Use rep max (RM) to guide rest times: Align your rest periods with intensity. For instance:
    - 5RM: Opt for about 5 minutes of rest between sets.
    - 5-7RM: 3-5 minutes of rest between sets.
    - 8-10RM: 2-3 minutes of rest between sets.
    - 11-13RM: 1-2 minutes of rest between sets.
    - Beyond 13RM: 30 seconds to one minute of rest between sets.

- Listen to your body: Pay attention to how your body feels during different rest intervals. Adjust based on your ability to perform each set with optimal effort and technique.

- Balance fatigue and recovery: The aim is to minimize fatigue at the start of each set by allowing sufficient recovery. This balance enables you to express strength effectively in each set.

By thoughtfully adjusting rest periods between sets, you can tailor your workout to suit your specific goals, whether they are focused on strength, power, stamina, or a combination of these elements. This customization ensures that each aspect of your workout is contributing effectively to your overall fitness progress.

Variable #7 - Tempo

Tempo refers to the speed at which you perform the repetitions of an exercise. Typically, this includes the concentric contraction (lifting and shortening phase of the exercise) and the eccentric contraction (lowering and lengthening phase of the exercise). For instance, as you lower toward the floor during a push up, the pecs lengthen and control the speed of your descent (i.e. eccentric contraction). As you push back up again, they shorten (i.e. concentric contraction).

Adjusting tempo of reps influences several key factors in your workout like muscle time under tension, power output, and neuromuscular control. A slower tempo increases the time your muscles are under tension, which can lead to increased hypertrophy (muscle growth). On the other hand, a faster tempo, particularly in the concentric phase, can enhance power and explosive strength.

Manipulating tempo can also be a strategic tool for overcoming weaknesses or limitations. For example, if you struggle with pull ups, emphasizing the eccentric (or lowering) phase of the exercise can help address the particular weak links to eventually perform full reps.

How to select the right tempo

- Understand general recommendations: A common tempo recommendation is 1 second for the concentric (or lifting) phase of an exercise and 1-3 seconds for the eccentric (or lowering) phase. However, this can vary based on the particular exercise and your specific goals.

- Use negatives for strength building: You are stronger during the eccentric phase of any exercise—as much as 1.75x stronger than the concentric phase. So if you're currently unable to do a single push-up, then focusing on the eccentric phase with a slower tempo (6-10 seconds) is effective at building the necessary strength towards full reps.

- Adjust tempo for power movements: For exercises requiring explosive power, like high pull ups, train the concentric phase more explosively. This trains your muscles to generate more force quickly.

- Consider muscle growth and endurance: Slower reps can be beneficial for hypertrophy and muscular endurance. Super slow training, where the tempo is 10 seconds on the way down and 10 seconds on the way up, can be particularly effective for muscle growth.

- Tailor tempo to your experience level: Begin learning new movements with a slower tempo to ensure proper technique and neuromuscular control. As you gain proficiency, increasing tempo can build power and challenge.

- Balance strength and power development: Prioritize developing strength before focusing on power. For example, progress to clapping push-ups only after you've developed sufficient wrist strength and can comfortably perform standard push-ups.

- Be mindful of movement patterns: Ensure that tempo adjustments don't compromise your form and technique. Maintaining control throughout the entire range of motion for an exercise is crucial, regardless of the tempo.

By manipulating the tempo of your repetitions, you tailor your workout to target specific aspects of fitness, whether it's building muscle, developing explosive power, or enhancing endurance. Tempo adjustment allows you to fine-tune each exercise to meet your unique goals and overcome personal challenges.

Variable #8 - Frequency

Frequency is the number of times that you exercise within a given time frame, typically measured on a weekly basis. This variable is crucial because it balances training with recovery.

The right frequency is vital for allowing adequate muscle and nervous system recovery. When frequency is too high, it can lead to overtraining where the body isn't able to recover between sessions. And when frequency is too low, progress can be too slow. The optimal frequency varies based on several factors like your current level, the intensity and volume of your workouts, and your body's individual recovery capacity.

How to Select the Right Frequency

- Assess your level: Beginners, who are still adapting their muscular and nervous systems to bodyweight exercises, may require longer recovery time than advanced practitioners. This should be reflected in a lower training frequency.

- Consider muscle recovery: Muscle recovery is an individual process. Pay attention to how your body feels in the days after your workout and adjust frequency accordingly. If you feel fatigued or sore, it is a sign to allow more recovery time.

- Balance intensity with frequency: Generally, the higher the intensity of your workouts, the lower your training frequency should be because high-intensity sessions require longer recovery times.

- Avoid overtraining: Be wary of the temptation to train excessively. High intensity training at a frequency of 5-6 sessions per week can interfere with your body's ability to recover.

- Incorporate active recovery: On days you're not strength training, consider engaging in activities that focus on mobility, stability, or light cardio. These activities aid in recovery and help develop other aspects of fitness without overtraining your muscles.

- Listen to your body: The most crucial aspect of determining the right frequency is to listen to your body's cues. Adapt and modify your training frequency based on your personal recovery needs and progress.

- Stay flexible and adaptive: As you progress in your fitness journey, your capacity for recovery may improve, allowing for increased frequency. Be open to adjusting your routine as your fitness level improves.

By adjusting the frequency of your workouts, you create a training schedule that maximizes effectiveness while respecting your body's need for rest and recovery. This approach ensures sustainable progress and reduces the risk of injury or burnout.

Crafting Your Unique Blueprint

In our journey through this chapter, we've unraveled a critical understanding: The pursuit of physical excellence is deeply personal and requires a custom-tailored approach. Just as our fingerprints are unique, so too are the paths we must walk in our fitness journey. There is no universal solution, no one-size-fits-all routine that can bring out the best in everyone.

As we conclude this exploration of constructing your personalized workout routine, remember that the design of every workout is a crucial component of an effective fitness program. Your goals are the compass that guide how you adjust various training variables to optimize your results. Each aspect — from the choice of exercises, their order, the intensity, number of sets, rest periods, tempo of repetitions, to the frequency of your workouts — must be carefully considered and tailored to your unique needs and objectives. This personalized approach ensures that your training is not just a series of exercises, but a strategic and effective path towards your goals.

Recall the story we started with — our community member who followed a generic routine from an influencer and hit a wall in his training. His experience underlines a critical truth in fitness that blindly following cookie-cutter plans leads to suboptimal results or even setbacks. His journey, much like yours, requires a routine that is customized, taking into account individual strengths, weaknesses, and specific aspirations.

Now, having equipped you with the tools to construct a routine as unique as your DNA, we turn towards the horizon of goal-setting—a crucial component in your expedition. The upcoming chapter introduces you to the most potent goal-setting framework known to man. This framework isn't just about setting targets; it's about architecting your ambitions into tangible realities. As you close this chapter and prepare to flip the page, you stand at the cusp of transforming the vision of your new physique from a distant dream into your present truth, all in the swiftest timeline that dedication and strategy can draw.

The process of adjusting these eight variables to suit your specific situation can be complicated, but don't get caught up in perfectionism. Just get started and then adjust along the way based on your experience. And get help if you need it.

Chapter Takeaways

- There is no such thing as the 'best' workout routine; there is only such a thing as the best workout routine for you.

- The eight training variables are like dials you can adjust to create a routine that suits your specific situation.

- The particular exercises you select (variable #1) and the order in which you perform them (variable #2) are the most important aspects of your routine.

- The number of sets you perform for each exercise (variable #3) at a certain level of intensity (variable #4) for a specific amount of reps (variable #5) will determine the total volume of your workout (volume = sets x intensity x reps).

- The length of rest periods you choose to take between sets (variable #6) will impact different dimensions of your fitness. For example, shorter rest periods can lead to better improvements in stamina while longer rest periods can lead to better improvements in strength and power.

- The tempo at which you perform your reps (variable #7) will impact how much time under tension your muscles accumulate. For beginners, a longer tempo makes sense because it helps develop mind-muscle connection. For advanced trainees, a shorter tempo can work better when developing power and explosiveness.

- How many times you choose to workout per week (variable #8) will impact how well your body recovers between sessions.

CHAPTER 12 - OKR GOAL SETTING

"If you go to work on your goals, your goals will go to work on you. If you go to work on your plan, your plan will go to work on you. Whatever good things we build end up building us."

—JIM ROHN

At the break of dawn, a man stands alone on a rooftop overlooking the empty streets below. His gaze is not on the fading stars but on the invisible horizon, the boundary of his ambition. This moment, under the cloak of a predawn shadow, is more than ritual—it's a statement and reaffirmation of the goals that drive him. Each silent breath is a commitment, a personal contract signed with the rising sun that he will pursue his potential no matter what.

Goals are the silent warriors in the conquest of self. They are the challenges we set not in the light of day but in the solitude of introspection, where our true desires reveal themselves. But it's not our aim alone that carves the path to success; it is our discipline and commitment to the process.

Consider that the champion and the contender both desire victory. But desire without direction is like an arrow without a target. What separates a fleeting wish from a tangible triumph is laser-focused clarity of purpose coupled with carefully crafted daily habits.

In this chapter we dive into the world of Objectives and Key Results (OKRs) – a powerful goal-setting framework that has driven the success of global giants like Google, Microsoft and Netflix. But OKRs are not confined to the boardrooms of industry leaders; they are a tool for anyone daring to dream boldly and seeking to bring those dreams into reality.

In the following pages, we will deconstruct the essence of OKR goal setting, tailoring its methodology to your personal fitness journey. This is not just about goal setting; it's about revolutionizing the way you approach your aspirations by aligning your daily actions with your ultimate objectives.

Prepare to embark on a transformative journey where your fitness goals go from being silent thoughts in your mind to becoming the driving force of your daily life.

The Foundation Of Okrs

OKRs, standing for objective and key results, represents a multi-faceted goal management system. First, it is a powerful way to formulate your strategy with clear, measurable and action oriented objectives. And second, the system guides the implementation and execution of your personalized strategy. OKRs are not just about establishing targets; they're about aligning your daily behaviors and actions with the results that matter most. The framework consists of three core elements:

1. **Objective:** An objective describes where you want to go and sets a clear direction. Think of it like a certain destination or point on a map. Objectives should be

inspirational and understandable without technical jargon or metrics. An objective answers the question: "Where do I want to go?"

2. **Key Results:** A key result shows you how you are progressing towards your objective. Think of these like signposts with a distance marker telling you if you're getting closer to the objective or not. Key results answer the question: "How do I know if I'm getting to where I want to go?"

3. **Initiatives:** An initiative describes what you'll do to influence your key results. Think of it as the description of the actions you'll take to get to your desired destination. Initiatives answer the question: "What will I do to get to where I want to go?"

To explain OKRs through a metaphor, imagine setting out on a road trip. Your objective is the destination (let's say Los Angeles), key results are the signposts indicating distance and direction, and initiatives are the practical steps (e.g. fueling up, checking tire pressure, getting a good night's sleep) ensuring that you reach your goal.

The power of OKRs lies in their ability to make your strategy clear and actionable. They prioritize the actions with the most significant impact on your objectives, giving you measurable outcomes to focus on what truly matters.

By setting OKRs, you're not just dreaming; you're doing. This framework helps you prioritize and focus on what truly moves the needle in your fitness (and life). It's not a set-and-forget system; it's dynamic, requiring regular check-ins and fine-tuning. This continuous loop of evaluation and improvement means you don't just reach your goals; you expand and evolve them.

Example Of Okrs In Fitness

Objective:

- Live a long and healthy life

Key Results:

- Decrease waist measurement from 40 to 32 inches
- Increase pull up strength from 5 to 10 full reps
- Increase VO_2 max from 30 to 50

Initiatives:

- Construct a weekly nutrition plan
- Practice time-restricted eating by fitting all meals between 10am-6pm
- Walk 10,000 steps daily
- Workout 3 times per week
- Build an excel spreadsheet to track workout progress
- Get to bed by 10:30pm every single night on weekdays
- Go on 90 minute hike every Saturday morning
- Ride bike to work on Mondays, Wednesdays and Fridays.
- Practice breathwork as part of morning routine

Writing Effective Okrs

The way you articulate your OKRs can dramatically influence their effectiveness. Well-written OKRs inspire and guide you, but poorly constructed ones can destroy your motivation.

- Types of Objectives: These can be to 'build' (create something new), 'improve' (enhance something existing), or 'innovate' (completely reinvent).

- Key Results: Should be outcome-focused and have a clear metric. They should stretch your abilities without breaking them, balancing ambition with realism.

- Initiatives: Must be specific, action-oriented, and within your control. They directly influence your key results.

Structure them with clear action verbs.

Whether you're starting a fitness journey, improving your routine, or reinventing your approach, your OKRs should reflect your personal fitness narrative.

Your Path To Mastery

Remember, OKRs are not about reaching a destination and calling it quits; they're about journeying to a place where you want to live, grow, and continue to set new horizons. As you learn to integrate OKRs into your life, you'll find that the clarity they provide in your quest for fitness can be applied to any area —career, personal development, relationships—propelling you toward a future of your own deliberate design.

In the beginning of this chapter, we joined an athlete at the starting line, his entire journey ahead was based on the clarity of his vision and precision of his goals. Much like our athlete setting his sights on the finish line, you've now charted your course with OKRs, transforming abstract aspirations into tangible targets. But OKRs are more than just signposts on your journey to health and vitality; they are commitments that tell a narrative in which you are the man in the arena rather than a spectator on the sidelines.

As you progress, remember that your journey is about more than just the goals you reach; it's about the mindset you cultivate along the way. This isn't about a temporary change or a quick fix. It's about a fundamental transformation in how you view yourself. The next chapter will dive into the core of this mentality. You'll learn how to cultivate a mindset that remains unphased by setbacks and is actually fueled by them—a mindset that doesn't rely on bursts of motivation but is powered by ingrained habits and a deep-seated commitment to continual improvement.

So as we transition from the tactical structure of OKRs, let's pave the way to understanding the psychology upon which these frameworks rest. We'll explore how to integrate your goals into your very being so that the pursuit of health and fitness is not just something you do, but a defining part of who you are.

Prepare to dive into the Mastery Mentality, a powerful ally that will ensure the permanence of your success. It's the force that keeps your momentum going even when the initial excitement wears off. With this mentality, you'll learn how to stick to the process, weather the storms of challenge, and celebrate the spectrum of small victories on the long road to achieving your grandest goals.

Chapter Takeaways

- Objectives and Key Results (OKRs) are a practical and effective framework for setting and achieving goals. This framework, used by successful companies like Google and Microsoft, is adaptable for our personal fitness journey.

- Articulating OKRs effectively, with different types of objectives (build, improve, innovate), outcome-focused key results, and specific, action-oriented initiatives is the key to making them work for you.

- OKRs are not a one-time achievement but a continuous process of setting, achieving, and evolving goals. This concept applies not just to fitness but to all areas of life.

CHAPTER 13 - THE MASTERY MENTALITY

"We fail to realize that mastery is not about perfection. It's about a process, a journey. The master is the one who stays on the path day after day, year after year. The master is the one who is willing to try, and fail, and try again, for as long as he or she lives."

—GEORGE LEONARD

He hangs from the pullup bar, muscles tensed, mind focused. Each movement is deliberate, each breath a silent mantra of the progress he seeks. The cold metal against his palms is less an obstacle and more a familiar challenge, one that whispers tales of the slow, transformative journey of mastery that lies ahead.

Mastery in the realm of calisthenics is a mysterious dance where the dynamics of movement and the rhythm of practice merge into an art form. The road to mastery is less about arrival and more about continuous growth and improvement. It's the subtle shift from unlocking your first pull up to the exploration of your body's limitless capacity for movement through space.

The path of mastery stretches out with each new exercise mastered and each limitation overcome. This path is not marked by the quick wins that often fade as quickly as they arrive, but by the persistent, incremental gains that compound over time. On this journey, the distance between knowledge and action narrows until they move in harmony.

Embracing the Mastery Mentality in calisthenics means acknowledging that with every new feat accomplished, the landscape of what's possible expands. As your skills grow, the path ahead unfolds, offering endless potential for those willing to pursue the course.

In this chapter, we dive into the heart of the Mastery Mentality and how it contrasts from the Dabbler's approach—one being a sustainable pursuit that becomes part of who you are, and the other being a quick sprint with no lasting victory.

In the context of calisthenics, adopting a Mastery Mentality is about embracing the beauty of the basics and the complex alike. It's about seeing the grand potential in every push up, the foundational strength in every hollow body hold, and the incremental victories in every second held in a handstand.

The Five Tenets Of Mastery

Throughout this chapter, we'll explore how the Mastery Mentality transcends the physical practice and becomes a cornerstone of one's character. It's about pursuing improvement not just for the sake of mastery itself, but for the personal evolution it represents.

You'll learn why this mindset is crucial for long-term progress and how it can be nurtured day by day. By the end, you'll have a map to guide you along the path of calisthenics mastery, ensuring that each step you take is purposeful and each milestone, a marker of the strength within.

Tenet #1 - Delay Immediate Gratification

In the pulsating rhythm of our modern world, we are pulled by the siren song of immediate gratification, instant success, and quick fixes. This song is tempting, but it can lead us astray into a mirage of fleeting achievements. Our society is trapped in the quicksand of consumerism, where the appeal of the immediate overshadows the beauty of the enduring.

Our attraction to the immediate is something we evolved with. Our ancestors, living under the harsh conditions of the primal world, were attuned to the urgent needs of the moment – a chase for the next meal, getting away from immediate danger, or finding shelter against the approaching storm. In those times, prioritizing the moment was not just practical; it was existential. Our brains, sculpted by the hands of evolution, became wired to favor instant rewards over long-term results.

Yet, we find ourselves in a different world. The modern landscape, with its technological advancements and societal complexities, demands a different approach. It is here that the first tenet of the Mastery Mentality whispers its timeless wisdom:

Delaying gratification in the short-term is necessary for enjoying greater rewards in the long-term.

This tenet is not just a strategy; it is a philosophy, a way of life that promotes the virtue of patience and the fulfillment of gradual, sustained progress.

Picture two men embarking on their fitness journey – a newcomer and a veteran. The newcomer, filled with enthusiasm, leaps into advanced techniques but his body is unprepared for the demands of such intensity. His technique is haphazard and his joints take a beating. Each session presents a new challenge as he dances with the enticing illusion of rapid progress.

The veteran approaches his training with a different mindset. Day after day, he sticks to his routine, incrementally pushing his boundaries, resisting the seductive pull of instant success. His progress is not drastic; it's gradual, almost imperceptible. But it is real, tangible, and sustainable. Months pass, and the story unfolds predictably – the newcomer, consumed by his pursuit of the immediate, burns out, gets injured, and gives up. The veteran shows up day by day, getting stronger with his skills honed by the wisdom of patience and persistence.

This tale is a parable of mastery. The veteran, with his commitment to the long game, understands that true progress, the kind that lasts, is experienced over time. In resisting the siren call of instant gratification, the master lays a foundation for achievements that are not just impressive, but also lasting.

Delaying gratification is essential for long-term success. It guides us to look beyond the immediacy of the now so that we can match our behaviors in the moment with our objectives for the future. In the heart of this tenet lies the secret to not just achieving mastery, but living it.

Tenet #2 - Learn To Love The Process

Those who thirst for immediate success find themselves stuck in a perpetual cycle of fleeting victories. Results that come easy leave the exact same way. The path of mastery requires something different and is not for the faint of heart. This path demands a commitment to the process – a journey filled with practice, perseverance, and patience.

Think of painting a timeless piece of art, brushstroke by brushstroke, with each layer of paint representing hours of dedication. It is in these hours of seemingly mundane practice and drudgery that the seeds of true achievement are sown. The process is often invisible to the outside world, but it is the crucible in which mastery is forged.

In a world obsessed with results, being process-oriented is a quiet rebellion, a path less traveled. It is a journey that demands focus on the incremental steps that lie in front of you. Mastery is not about reaching a destination; it is about falling in love with the process. When you learn to love the process, consistency becomes an ally, and results become a natural consequence rather than an obsessive pursuit.

Consider the tale of two individuals learning the handstand. One is obsessed with achieving the perfect handstand, each fall is seen as a failure with frustration resulting from every tumble. The other, however, immerses himself in the nuances of the journey – the alignment, the core engagement, the delicate balance. This individual is not untouched by failure but views each attempt as an opportunity to learn, adapt, and improve. Through the passage of time, the one who embraced the process not only achieves the handstand but also revels in the richness of the journey. The results-oriented individual, meanwhile, has already abandoned the quest, overwhelmed by frustration and impatience.

The master understands that the process is within his control but results are not. By valuing the process, every loss is transformed into a lesson and every challenge is seen as an opportunity for growth. With a fixation on results, failure is perceived as defeat, not realizing that in pursuit of mastery, each thread of experience contributes to the magnificent final picture.

The second tenet of the Mastery Mentality is to shift your gaze from the distant horizon of results to the rich landscape of the process. For it is in this landscape that the true essence of mastery blooms – not in the fleeting glow of achievement, but in the enduring light of growth and learning.

Tenet #3 - Get Laser Focused

With access to the internet comes access to all of human information at our fingertips at the speed of light. Glued to our screens, we are bombarded by distractions that glitter with promises and each scroll reveals another tempting possibility. It is in this whirlwind of choices that the true challenge of mastery reveals itself as the art of focus.

> *"In an information-rich world, the wealth of information means a dearth of something else: a scarcity of whatever it is that information consumes. What information consumes is rather obvious: it consumes the attention of its recipients. Hence a wealth of information creates a poverty of attention and a need to allocate that attention efficiently among the overabundance of information sources that might consume it."*
>
> **—Herbert A. Simon**

The fact that you've made it to the final chapter of this book means that you are a rare individual that is committed to making a change. But stay wary of tomorrow's temptations - a different training style on Instagram, a new fitness trend on social media, an ad for a breakthrough piece of equipment. These distractions dangle just within our reach, yet escape our grasp at the last moment.

The master navigates this world with a different compass. He has his blinders on and remains laser-focused on his chosen path, ignoring the siren calls that beckon from every corner. Distractions are an ever-present, ever-growing tempest in our journey, but the master exerts his will to manage them and remains steadfast in his pursuit.

Consider the story of Odysseus and how he protected himself and his crew from being distracted by the Siren's song. In the story, Sirens are mythical creatures with the bodies of birds and the heads of women. They are known for their enchanting and irresistible song that lures sailors to their doom. According to the myth, any sailor who hears the Sirens' song becomes hypnotized, loses all sense of reason and is drawn towards the source of the song, often leading to their ships being wrecked on the rocky coast where the Sirens reside.

As Odysseus and his crew are about to pass the Sirens' island, he is warned about the danger of the Sirens' song. Odysseus heeds the warning and orders his men to plug their ears with beeswax so that they would not be able to hear the Sirens. However, Odysseus, curious to hear the Sirens' song himself without falling into the trap, instructs his men to tie him securely to the ship's mast and orders them not to untie him, no matter how much he begs and orders them to do so.

As they sail past the island, the Sirens start singing their bewitching song. Odysseus, upon hearing it, is instantly captivated and pleads with his men to release him, but they obey his original orders and sail past the island safely. This ancient story echoes the timeless truth of protecting ourselves against the seduction of distraction.

The story of Odysseus illustrates the essence of the third tenet of mastery. The master takes proactive measures to avoid getting distracted. Mastery means committing to a chosen strategy and seeing it through to fruition. In contrast, the dabbler is swayed by the currents of superficial trends, hopping from one approach to another, yet advancing little in any. The master has a clear understanding of his own journey and isn't distracted by every trend because he knows that meaningful results are achieved through focused effort over time.

Tenet #4 - Dive Deep

In pursuit of mastery, we must dive deep. To stay on the surface is to be deceived by the appearance of the tip of the iceberg. True mastery, much like the submerged foundation of the iceberg, dwells in the depths that escape the casual observer's eye.

The ease with which a master executes a skill is what we see. What we don't see is the countless years of deliberate practice dedicated to his craft.

Consider the Chinese bamboo. The bamboo seed lies dormant under the soil, showing no sign of life for five years. It is a period of unseen activity, where an intricate and vast network of roots spreads silently in the depths of the earth. This stage, often mistaken for inactivity, is the bamboo's deep-rooted commitment to growth. Then, in an astonishing burst of life, the bamboo shoots up to an astounding ninety feet in just a few weeks. This rapid growth seems sudden on the surface but it is actually the result of five years of patient and persistent construction of its deep foundations.

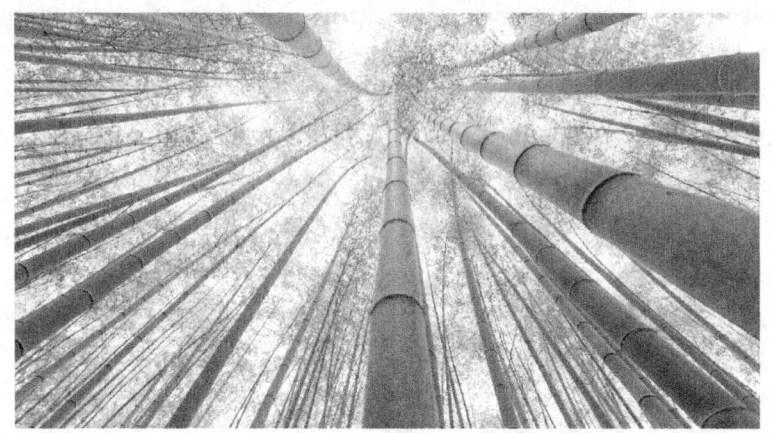

The Chinese bamboo grows a couple of inches in its first five years before shooting up to ninety feet within six weeks.

The growth of Chinese bamboo mirrors the journey of mastery. On the surface, progress may seem slow, almost non-existent, much like the bamboo in its initial years. Yet, beneath the surface, there is a deep foundation being established. To the uninitiated, the master's ease of execution appears supernatural, but it is the visible expression of years of dedicated, unseen practice.

Let us revisit the park where two individuals practice pull ups. One attempts the exercise as a routine task, ignoring proper technique but counting reps and sets, much like a farmer who impatiently checks for sprouts without nurturing the soil. The other, like the gardener who patiently tends to the bamboo, immerses in the depth of the exercise. Every grip, every tempo, every movement is an exploration, an opportunity to strengthen the foundation of their skill. This individual understands that mastery, like the bamboo, requires a deep, invisible network of dedication and insight, which, when the time is right, propels growth that is both rapid and astonishing.

The dabbler, who only counts reps, is like a gardener fixated on the barren surface, unaware of the potential that lies in the depths. In contrast, the master is like the bamboo farmer, who knows that true growth, true mastery, is a process of nurturing the roots – the unseen, the intricate, the profound.

The fourth tenet of the Mastery Mentality invites us to embrace the wisdom of the Chinese bamboo. It encourages us to focus on building a deep, extensive foundation, understanding that visible progress is but a reflection of the depth of our unseen work. The heights we reach depend on the depths we explore and the roots we establish. It is in this depth that the heart and soul of mastery lives, waiting to burst forth in its own perfect time.

Tenet #5 - Commit Wholeheartedly

In the quest for mastery, consistent action is just the beginning. The spirit with which one engages in the pursuit is what truly defines the journey. The fifth tenet of the Mastery Mentality speaks to the heart of commitment – the difference between simply showing up and being fully present in the moment. It's about the quality of attention and intensity of purpose that one brings to their practice.

Imagine two friends working out together. One immerses himself in each movement, every rep is a moment of connection and dialogue between body and mind. He is focused and present with a clear intention – he is not just going through the motions, he is going for mastery. The other friend, however, is only half there; his attention is split between the workout and his phone, his movements lack conviction and his mind is wandering. This dichotomy between wholehearted and half-hearted commitment defines our fifth tenet. Over time, the difference in their approaches create very different outcomes.

The wholehearted practitioner experiences transformation, not just in physical form, but in mental and emotional realms as well. Each workout becomes more than a physical activity; it becomes a medium for personal growth, a space for cultivating discipline, focus, and character. The master, in his wholehearted approach, finds that his practice enriches not just his body, but his entire being.

In contrast, the half-hearted practitioner, distracted and disengaged, finds little satisfaction or progress. His approach is like skimming the surface of a vast ocean – never diving deep enough to discover the treasures that lie beneath. He may be showing up, but he is not evolving. The dabbler, in his lack of commitment, misses the essence of the journey and the transformative power of a practice that is embraced with one's whole heart.

The fifth tenet of the Mastery Mentality is about committing wholeheartedly to our pursuits. It is a call to be present, observant, and curious in our journey towards mastery. It is a reminder that the way we engage in our practice reflects the way we engage in life. The master knows that half-hearted efforts yield half-hearted results. True mastery, therefore, is not just about the actions we take but about the heart and soul we pour into them. It is about bringing our full presence and commitment to each moment, embracing the journey with an open mind.

Tenet #6 - Enlist Support

The master understands that lasting achievement is rarely a solo performance. This understanding forms the cornerstone of the sixth tenet of the Mastery Mentality that recognizes the journey to excellence as a path best traveled with allies, mentors, and comrades.

The master knows that the lone wolf is a vulnerable creature. In the harsh realities of nature, when the cold winds blow, it's the pack that survives. The lone wolf may roam with a semblance of freedom, but in times of trial, it's the strength of the pack that endures. This wisdom translates seamlessly into our quest for mastery. The master doesn't stand alone; he stands on the shoulders of those who support him, understanding that in collaboration lies strength.

Looking back to the ancient story of Odysseus, he knew the limitations of human willpower. He didn't rely solely on his own discipline to resist temptation. Instead, he enlisted the support of his crew. He had them fill their ears with beeswax and instructed his men to tie him securely to the ship's mast, ensuring that no matter how beguiled he became, he would not give in to the Sirens' call. Odysseus's story teaches us that sometimes, the greatest strength lies in recognizing our own vulnerabilities and proactively seeking support.

This understanding that we are stronger together is not just intuitive but empirically proven. Patients that underwent heart bypass surgery were told by doctors that they needed to make significant changes in their lifestyle. Otherwise, their time on this planet would end a lot sooner than it had to. In looking at the data, Dr. Edward Miller, dean of Johns Hopkins Medical

School and CEO of the John Hopkins Medical Center, tells us that:

"If you look at people after coronary-artery bypass grafting two years later, 90% of them have not changed their lifestyle."

Faced with the imminent threat of death, an overwhelming majority still fail to change their choices[9]. But there was another group of patients that had a much higher success rate. This group met regularly to share their experiences, challenges, and progress. The result was a success rate of nearly 80%. Contrast this with the group attempting to make changes on their own that had a success rate of 10%. The lesson is that if you're attempting to make a change, don't go it alone.

In our coaching program, this principle of support is a fundamental pillar. Many clients join us claiming that their biggest struggle is staying consistent. But when we get them into our system, all of a sudden they haven't missed a single workout in an entire year. This isn't the case with every client of course, but it's my observation that accountability is often the bridge between intention and execution. Look back to your own past efforts at making changes in your lifestyle. Did those changes stick? If not, did you enlist support?

The sixth tenet of the Mastery Mentality is a reminder on the power of the pack. The master knows that nothing great is ever achieved alone. The lone wolf may roam, but it is within the pack that true strength, endurance, and success are found.

Step away from the myth of solitary conquest and join a community of support. Whether it's through our coaching program, friends, family, or a local fitness community, the key is to connect, to get accountable, and to grow together.

What Path Will You Choose

As we near the end of this transformative journey through the world of calisthenics and the Mastery Mentality, let's revisit the vivid imagery we started with - the focused athlete hanging from the pull up bar. This image is a metaphor for the journey you, the reader, have embarked upon. Each tenet explored in this chapter makes up the mindset you must have on this path to mastery, a path that requires more than physical strength; it demands mental resilience, emotional intelligence, and a soulful commitment to growth.

These tenets are not just strategies; they are principles that transcend the realm of fitness and seep into the very fabric of our lives. They are the cornerstones of a Mastery Mentality, guiding us to not only pursue mastery in calisthenics but to embrace it as a cornerstone of our character, reshaping our bodies, our minds, and our lives.

As we transition from this chapter to the conclusion of our book, we carry with us the essence of these tenets. The final chapter is not an end but a beginning – the start of your lifelong journey towards calisthenics mastery. We will reflect on all that we've learned, tying together the threads of knowledge and insight into a cohesive tapestry. This journey, much like our opening scene of the athlete on the pullup bar, is about continuous growth and improvement, exploring the vast potential of the human spirit.

In the conclusion, we will synthesize the insights gained, offering a holistic view of how the Mastery Mentality can transform your approach to fitness and your approach to life. We'll provide the final pieces of the puzzle, leaving you equipped and inspired to continue your journey long after the last page is turned. Prepare for the last leg of this journey, where we bring together all the elements of mastery, setting the stage for a lifetime of growth, exploration, and progress.

Chapter Takeaways

- Like the veteran who resists the lure of quick fixes, patience and persistence are the keys that unlock true progress in fitness and in life.

- When you learn to love the process, the results take care of themselves.

- The tale of Odysseus teaches the importance of staying true to our chosen path, avoiding the distractions that lead us astray.

- The Chinese bamboo metaphor illustrates the necessity of cultivating a deep foundation, ensuring that our growth, when it comes, is both rapid and sustainable.

- Through the contrasting approaches of two friends, we've grasped the significance of engaging with our whole heart, making every rep, every moment count.

CONCLUSION - THE PATH AHEAD

"Though no one can go back and make a brand-new start, anyone can start from now and make a brand-new ending."

—CARL BARD

Imagine standing at a crossroads, the path behind you worn with your footsteps, reflecting the journey you've just taken through the pages of this book. Each chapter was a step, some challenging, others enlightening, but all leading to this moment of realization.

You've traveled through the rugged terrain of fitness, soared on the winds of calisthenics mastery, and navigated the twists and turns of mental fortitude. Now, as you pause here, you face the path ahead with a new perspective—a path of strength, health, and vitality that you carve with every choice from this day forward.

To recap what we've covered:

1. In the first few chapters of this book, we took a deep dive into the Holy Grail of fitness which we defined as

longevity—living a long and healthy life.

We discussed the unique advantages of bodyweight exercise in the context of longevity and also where calisthenics falls short when it comes to lower-body development.

2. Next, we looked at the multiple dimensions of fitness and how bodyweight exercise can help us develop all of them at the same time.

We looked at your current levels of fitness across the multiple dimensions, what areas needed improving, and even broke down your current versus optimal physique proportions based on the Golden Ratio.

We also deconstructed the universal Laws of Lifting so that your approach to fitness can be anchored in timeless principles without being swayed by the latest fads.

3. In Creating Alignment Parts I & II, we looked at how musculoskeletal alignment is the hidden key to long-term success in fitness.

We also explored the **Simple Six Exercises** and walked you through the **Bodyweight Fitness Standards** so that you can navigate your fitness journey with clarity.

4. In the final section of the book, we deconstructed the variables of personalized training that debunked the one-size-fits-all approach presenting you with a tailor-made suit of personal growth that is cut precisely for your individuality.

We looked at how to set goals using the Objectives and Key Results framework.

And last of all, we explored the **Mastery Mentality** and how to install a mindset that guarantees your success.

Now, with the book's mission laid out and each takeaway interwoven with the overarching theme, it's clear what the essence of this journey has been. It's about rejecting the appeal of quick fixes and embracing the enduring satisfaction of genuine progress. It's about looking past the shiny exterior of extreme diets and flashy workouts to discover the true nature of sustainable fitness—a harmony of body and mind, built to last a lifetime.

The next step for you is simple.

Start.

Decide if you want help or if you want to go it alone, but start. Make one small decision, then take the one small step in front of you.

Starting Calisthenics won't make you a functional athlete overnight, but it can increase your strength, mobility and physical capability over time—no matter your age or current situation.

First though, you have to start.

Download the implementation resources I've put together for you here: calisthenicsbook.com/bonus.

If you're committed to becoming more capable (not less) with age and looking for personal guidance on the path, I want to be the one to support you through the process.

Your journey continues.
MO SALEEM

ABOUT THE AUTHOR

Ex-bodybuilder turned calisthenics enthusiast, Mo Saleem is the founder of Calisthenics School and is on a mission to make bodyweight training the new norm in fitness. Before discovering the power of bodyweight exercise, Mo faced severe injuries in the gym, which became pivotal points leading to his exploration of a myriad of holistic health practices.

After healing without surgery, Mo started sharing his methods online and coached over 5,000 individuals to achieve their fitness goals and sustain injury-free lifestyles.

Mo enjoys training combat sports, going on adventurous hikes, playing intense games of ping pong, and reading books on spirituality and business.

Above all, Mo believes that family comes first and that fitness should be a tool for showing up with more energy and presence in the lives of those you love most. That includes serving as a strong role model for the next generation.

All inquiries for podcast appearances, video shows, and speaking can be sent to mo@mosaleem.com.

---

[1] Brito LB et al., "Ability to sit and rise from the floor as a predictor of all-cause mortality," *European Journal of Preventive Cardiology*, July 2014, available online at https://pubmed.ncbi.nlm.nih.gov/23242910/.

[2] World Health Organization. "Falls." *World Health Organization*, 26 April 2021, https://www.who.int/news-room/fact-sheets/detail/falls.

[3] Katzmarzyk, P.T., & Leon, A.S. "Targeting the Metabolic Syndrome with Exercise: Evidence from the HERITAGE Family Study." *The Journal*

of Applied Physiology, vol. 99, no. 3, 2005, pp. 1206-1213. National Center for Biotechnology Information, https://www.ncbi.nlm.nih.gov/pmc/articles/PMC2453303/.

[4] Haskell, W.L., et al. "Physical Activity and Public Health: Updated Recommendation for Adults from the American College of Sports Medicine and the American Heart Association." Circulation, vol. 116, no. 9, 2007, pp. 1081-1093. *National Center for Biotechnology Information,* https://www.ncbi.nlm.nih.gov/pmc/articles/PMC3098120/.

[5] Haskell, W.L., et al. "Physical Activity and Public Health: Updated Recommendation for Adults from the American College of Sports Medicine and the American Heart Association." Circulation, vol. 116, no. 9, 2007, pp. 1081-1093. *National Center for Biotechnology Information,* https://www.ncbi.nlm.nih.gov/pmc/articles/PMC3098120/.

[6] Fields KB. Running injuries - changing trends and demographics. *Curr Sports Med Rep* 2011; 10:299-303.

[7] Piercy, K.L., et al. "The Physical Activity Guidelines for Americans." *JAMA,* vol. 320, no. 19, 2018, pp. 2020-2028. National Center for Biotechnology Information, https://www.ncbi.nlm.nih.gov/pmc/articles/PMC6179786/.

[8] Sihvonen, R., et al. "Arthroscopic Partial Meniscectomy versus Sham Surgery for a Degenerative Meniscal Tear." *The New England Journal of Medicine,* vol. 369, no. 26, 2013, pp. 2515-2524. https://www.nejm.org/doi/full/10.1056/NEJMoa1305189.

[9] Alan Deutschman, "Change or Die," *Fast Company,* May 2005, available online at: https://www.fastcompany.com/677632/change-or-die-book-and-resolutions.